A GIFT FROM NATE

A story of a
Double Lung Transplant

Jay Crowley

In today's world, everything can be replaced, thank goodness!!

Thanks to people who shared their loved one's organs to help other families.

This story is dedicated to them.

Please become a donor.

The story is a partial work of non-fiction.

The places and events are real, but not all the people.

Some names and situations are products of the author's

imagination.

However, the transplant procedures, statistics and

terminology should be correct for that period of time.

Medical information for this book came from the

University of Colorado, the Mayo Clinic, Wikipedia and

medical web sites.

Please send an email: jaycrowleybooks@gmail.com

Your opinions of this story are welcome.

For updates on new stories and more information,

please visit www. sweetdreamsbooks.com

What happens in life is not always of your choosing. However, you adapt, as we are always in survival mode.

Jay Crowley

Table of Contents

PROLOG

I wrote this story for many reasons, one was we lived through this experience, so it is a healing process. Secondly, was to give the reader as much information in one spot as possible. Hopefully this will be helpful for people getting ready to go through the transplant procedure. Maybe this will answer some of their questions.

+++

The process of waiting and receiving a double lung transplant for my husband was a life changing experience for both of us. My husband was diagnosed with Idiopathic Pulmonary Fibrosis or IntralStatal disease in 2005. This story is about how our life went through so many emotions because of the illness being misdiagnosed, the waiting, the receiving, and the recovery of a double lung surgery. Then life after the necessary surgery. Below explains what causes a lung transplant to occur:

"Lung transplantation or pulmonary transplantation is a surgical procedure in which a patient's diseased lungs are partially or totally replaced by lungs which come from a donor. Donor lungs can be retrieved from a living donor or a deceased donor. With other lung diseases such as cystic fibrosis, it is imperative that a recipient receives two lungs. While lung transplants carry certain associated risks, they can also extend life expectancy and enhance the quality of life for end-stage pulmonary patients."

"Lung transplantation is the therapeutic measure of last resort for patients with end-stage lung disease who have exhausted all other available treatments without improvement. A variety of conditions may make such surgery necessary. As of 2005, the most common reasons for lung transplantation in the United States were:

27% chronic obstructive pulmonary disease (COPD), including emphysema;

16% idiopathic pulmonary fibrosis;

14% cystic fibrosis;

12% idiopathic (formerly known as "primary") pulmonary hypertension;

5% alpha 1-antitrypsin deficiency;

2% replacing previously transplanted lungs that have since failed.

24% other causes, including bronchiectasis and sarcoidosis."

Info from Stanford's Center for Advanced Lung Disease

Only about fifty-five percent of patients survive five years after the transplant. Those rates are better at some hospitals. However, only about two-thirds of patients can expect to survive that long. Nationwide, only a third of the patients live ten years, and it depreciates each year. It is unclear what, exactly, goes wrong after the first year. Most patients die of what is known as chronic rejection, which causes the airways of the lung to deteriorate slowly. Doctors don't know yet how to prevent or stop that process.

"I started doing (lung transplants) in the early '90s, and it was really primitive then, and it's gotten a lot better. All sorts of things have improved," said Dr. David Weill, director of Stanford's Center for Advanced Lung Disease. "But we haven't solved the mystery of that slow loss of lung function.

Fighting rejection after a lung transplant is an ongoing process. The body views the new lung, or lungs, as an invader and will continually attack it. (Stanford Center)

+++

I am not sure any of the information I have compiled in this is helpful to you, but I hope it is. I know when we started the process, I was trying to find information and was not sure where to look. You are dealing with new terminology and the whole transplant process. Here is some additional information.

"Before The Transplant; Entering the Transplant Program."

Their primary physician or specialist refers most candidates for transplantation to the program. Others come to be evaluated at their own initiative. The process begins with a call to the Lung Transplant Office. The patient will be asked to provide some basic medical information by telephone and to give us written permission to obtain medical records from other health care providers.

"Evaluation."

The common causes of lung failure that result in pulmonary transplantation are cystic fibrosis, emphysema (acquired, usually related to smoking; or resulting from an inherited protein abnormality: alpha-1 antitrypsin deficiency), idiopathic (otherwise unexplained) pulmonary fibrosis, and "primary" (otherwise unexplained) pulmonary hypertension. Together, these diagnoses account for about 9 of 10 lung transplant patients. A small percentage of patients who undergo pulmonary transplantation have venous vascular lung disease (disease of the blood vessels in the lungs), congenital lung disease (present at birth), or inoperable cardiac-related lung disease ("Eisenmenger's syndrome"), as the underlying condition.

"Which Procedure for Which Patient?"

For some patients, a single lung (one side, "single-lung transplant") is all that is needed. For others, both lungs ("double-lung transplant") or a heart as well as both lungs ("heart-lung transplant") are the best option. Occasionally, the decision about whether a given patient needs one lung or two will be influenced at the time of surgery, by the function of the donor, the availability of organs, or the severity illness of the recipient.

"Who Needs a Lung Transplant?"

In general, patients with advanced lung failure who continue to have severe symptoms (breathlessness with little or no exercise) on maximal medical therapy should be considered for transplant evaluation. In general, patients with increasing medication requirements, frequent hospitalizations, or overall deterioration of clinical status should be regarded as relatively urgent.

All candidates for transplantation begin the program with a comprehensive series of tests conducted by our multidisciplinary team of specialists. Some of these tests are required for any operative procedure (history and physical, chest X-ray, EKG, etc.) while others (such as special blood tests to learn about prior infection exposure) are required to optimize the recipient's care after the transplant.

During the evaluation, the lung transplant candidate will meet many members of the transplant team. Each member of the team will want to get to know the individual needing the transplant as well as all family members and friends who make up the candidate's health care and social support network. There are so many of us because a successful transplant program requires a combination of many people with different areas of expertise. While some aspects of transplantation have become routine, other aspects require innovation. This is where the experience of the team can make the difference between success and failure for an individual patient, particularly if the problem is unusual or severe. The various members of the team play different roles in each patient's care. During the evaluation phase, the candidate's primary contact person will be the transplant nurse practitioner.

Once the evaluation is complete, the transplant team will decide if a lung transplant is the best option. The risks and benefits will be discussed with each patient. If the patient and the transplant team agree that transplantation is the best available choice, the patient is then placed on the transplant waiting list at the University of Maryland Medical Center. This lung transplant waiting list is organized by the United Network for Organ Sharing (UNOS), which is the national list.

"What to Expect While Waiting"

The wait time may be short or long, depending on the donor supply and the patient waiting list. While waiting, the patient is seen in clinic periodically to assist with any medical issues that may arise. In addition to transplantation, patients with lung disease can be treated with various innovative and investigational modalities at the University of Maryland. The role of artificial lung support (also known as "ECMO," or extracorporeal membrane oxygenation) as a bridge to recovery or transplant is also being studied. Please remember that it is VERY IMPORTANT for the candidate and their physician to let us know promptly if there is any change in medication (especially steroid dose) or in the applicant's medical condition. When in doubt, CALL.

During the wait for a transplant, the primary contact person for medical problems will usually be the transplant pulmonologist. The transplant nurse practitioner or transplant secretary is always happy to field questions regarding transplantation.

"The Transplant"

When a compatible organ becomes available, the transplant patient is immediately contacted by a nurse coordinator and admitted to the hospital. At this time, a history is taken of any medical events, which may have occurred since the initial transplant evaluation. Appropriate testing is also done to ensure the patient's readiness for surgery.

Careful coordination is required between the donor and recipient surgical teams to minimize the amount of time that the new lung is "asleep." As soon as we are confident that the donor lung is in good condition and is suitable for the recipient, the patient is taken to the operating room. There, special IV lines are placed, and the recipient is carefully put to sleep by the anesthesia team. The chest is opened, and preparations are made to remove the old lung. Preparations may be made for supporting the recipient's circulation with a heart-lung ("cardiopulmonary bypass") machine if it appears that the circulation will not be adequate without this assistance.

Once the donor's lung has arrived safely, the old lung is removed, and the new lung stitched in place. This is done by sewing together the ends of the airway (bronchus) and main blood vessels (pulmonary artery and left atrium) leading in and out of the lung. After assuring that the new lung is working well, the chest is closed, leaving chest tubes to drain any blood or fluid that might otherwise accumulate around the new lung.

The surgery lasts approximately six to eight hours. When the operation is completed, the patient is taken to the intensive care unit. Over the subsequent days as the patient recovers from surgery, the breathing tube and various drainage tubes and intravenous lines are gradually removed, and the process of rehabilitation begins.

Occasionally the new lung may function poorly, due to unrecognized infection in the donor, or more commonly because of "ischemia/reperfusion injury." When this occurs, prolonged machine support using evolving lung ventilation strategies or even temporary artificial lung support (ECMO) may be required.

Careful, comprehensive post-surgical monitoring allows the

transplant team to continually evaluate whether the body is accepting the new organ. This includes regular lung X-rays, bronchoscopies, and periodic biopsies. Biopsies are performed through a bronchoscope inserted into the airway, and passing a delicate scissor device through the airway branches and into the lung under X-ray (fluoroscopy) guidance. Several small pieces of the lung are removed for microscopic examination.

The biopsy is essential: if we see evidence of immune injury to the lung (infiltration of cells called "lymphocytes"), then additional therapy may be prescribed to reverse this "acute rejection" process.

The average length of stay in the intensive care unit is 3-7 days, followed by 1-2 weeks in the hospital.

"After the Transplant/Going Home: The Outpatient Clinic"

Follow-up care initially involves returning to the Outpatient Clinic once a week for the first month after leaving the hospital. At this time a series of tests, including blood tests, are conducted to closely monitor the patient's progress. This is a period when medications are precisely adjusted. After this initial period of relatively intensive follow-up, patients are seen periodically as determined by their condition.

"The Patient's Responsibility"

While transplantation can significantly improve the quality of life of the recipients, it also demands much of them. They must become active participants in preserving their health.

"Immunosuppressive Medication"

Transplantation has become so successful in recent years in

large part through the development of new drugs, which prevent rejection of donated organs. These drugs inhibit the body's immune system from identifying the new organ as foreign. It is necessary for all patients to take immunosuppressive medication for the rest of their lives following transplant. A successful transplant can be undermined very quickly by the failure of patients to take their medications appropriately and responsibly.

Source: What to Expect Before, During and After the Lung Transplant | University of Maryland Medical Center."

Significant physiologic changes occur over the years following lung transplantation. Some changes affect all lung transplant recipients; others may be dependent upon the type of lung transplant surgery performed as in the case of double lung transplantation (BLT). The effect of lung transplantation is a long-term general respiratory physiology, in other words, you learn to live with it.

Lung transplantation alters many components of respiratory physiology. Some changes result from the surgical procedure, such as denervation of the transplanted lung, interrupted cough reflex, and reduced gastroesophageal motility. In other words, my husband, Cody has to force himself to cough. Nevertheless, regardless of the healing and emotional process, that lasts a lifetime, the transplant procedure is worth it. I hope that you will learn something about lung disease and the need for all types of transplants that may help you or a friend.

There are measures in place to help prevent the body from rejecting the organ. Immunosuppression drugs are prescribed to all transplant patients. Cody takes twenty-three meds a day. Medications such as corticosteroids and cyclosporine will be taken for the rest of his life to help suppress the immune system to keep the body from rejecting the organ. However, immune system-suppressing drugs also reduce the body's ability to fight off infections, so Cody has to take measures to avoid infection. Infections can be life threatening to him as he takes these immune suppressing drugs, specifically after an organ transplant. If the body rejects the new organ, death can result unless extensive measures, such as another transplant, can be done. In Cody case, he cannot receive another lung, as he is now too old. They do not like to perform a second lung transplant on a recipient over 65.

The words you dread to hear, you need a transplant: you think this couldn't possibly happen to us, or in many cases, when it does, wondering why us? However, no matter how bad things get during the transplant process, I want people to realize that you will survive anything to help your mate or family members in a health crisis. Hanging in there and supporting them is so important. Regardless of the flight or flight emotions that may occur.

I have tried to write this story as the process went along; it will reflect our anger, frustrations, and happiness. I tried not to dwell on the negative though it does have an effect on the process and our lives. The hardest part is learning "Nothing is the end of the world" and we can survive anything.

Throughout the process of illness, the family and the recipient have to cop an attitude. "God doesn't want me yet, and the Devil is afraid I will take over!"

+++

Our story is never ending as Cody is still alive and every day is an adventure now. He is eleven years out. However, now, about every six months, he has an episode of something; cold, virus, eyes, bones, or heart, but he is a fighter.

Best of all, I hope you will sign a donor card to save a person's life; you can do so at the Department of Motor Vehicles. **"Heaven doesn't need your organs, but heaven knows we need them here."** One donor can help hundred and fifty people.

Chapter One - In the Beginning

When Cody and I got married, it was the second marriage for both of us. Cody did not have any children, and I still had one child (out of four) still at home. Cody is a handsome, tall, slender man with cold eyes that can sparkle like diamonds. However, he was a glutton for punishment, marrying a woman with a teenager daughter. We both had good jobs, a nice home, so life was good. After the graduation of my youngest daughter, we bought a Recreational Vehicle to travel, as we both like to camp. Cody also liked to race a drag car, a 1971 Dodge Dart door-slammer, and the RV could house the crew. We were enjoying life.

In 1993 we purchased a 1968 Charger to show at car shows. Therefore, between working, having fun, and maintaining a couple acres of land, we were busy. We had a big garden, plus chickens, turkeys, and a Peacock. Urban farmers...

Cody worked shift work, usually grave or swing. I worked a sixty-plus hour a week job, but we had the weekends off. As stated, we both like to travel and love to go on ship cruises. We spent a lot of time at the National Hot Rod Association (NHRA) races. When Cody was not racing, he was working on the cars. So you can see we were people that love to live life, have fun and party. We never dreamed an illness could change our lives. Neither of us ever figured we would have so much drama in our lives in the years to follow.

+++

Our life did not change overnight. It took years. Early 2000, my 50 years old, husband, was diagnosed with COPD (Chronic Obstructive Pulmonary Disease). He was a smoker and had been for years. However, he also had been exposed to chemicals while in the military.

"COPD is a lung disease that makes it hard to breathe. It is caused by damage to the lungs over many years, usually from smoking. COPD is often a mix of two diseases:

Chronic bronchitis (say "bron-KY-tus"). In chronic bronchitis, the airways that carry air to the lungs (bronchial tubes camera.gif) get inflamed and make a lot of mucus. This can narrow or block the airways, making it hard for you to breathe.

Emphysema (say "em-fuh-ZEE-muh"). In a healthy person, the tiny air sacs in the lungs are like balloons. As you breathe in and out, they get bigger and smaller to move air through your lungs. However, with emphysema, these air sacs are damaged and lose their stretch. Less air gets in and out of the lungs, which makes you feel short of breath.

COPD gets worse over time. You cannot undo the damage to your lungs. However, you can take steps to prevent more damage and to feel better. What are the symptoms? The main symptoms are:

A long-lasting (chronic) cough.

Mucus that comes up when you cough.

Shortness of breath that gets worse when you exercise.

As COPD gets worse, you may be short of breath even when you do simple things like getting dressed or fixing a meal. It gets harder to eat or exercise, and breathing takes much more energy. People often lose weight and get weaker.

At times, your symptoms may suddenly flare up and get much worse. This is called a COPD exacerbation (say "egg-ZASS-er-BAY-shun"). An exacerbation can range from mild to life-threatening. The longer you have COPD, the more severe these flare-ups will be." *Info from **Medical MD off the internet.***

+++

When Cody became very ill, he went on sick leave. He had never been sick in fifteen years, so thank goodness, he had over nine months of sick and vacation leave to use.

His primary Doctor was not sure exactly what was wrong with Cody. Nevertheless, the Doctor placed him on inhalers and treated him as if he had emphysema. Also, he referred him to a group of respiratory specialists in Reno.

We live in rural Nevada, so our medical care is limited. To receive decent medical care, you must travel to Reno, Las Vegas or out of state. When Cody became sick over seventeen years ago, we had a shortage of specialized doctors, in fact, any doctors period. It was an interesting time for individuals with a significant illness.

+++

While in the Air Force. Cody was stationed in Arizona in a Titian II missile silo, during the Cold War. A rocket leaked, and the whole crew was exposed to missile fuel. Also, the silo was built with asbestos.

The Doctors in Reno never once took this into consideration; their first thought was COPD because he smoked.

However, after six months of seeing these specialists and their treatment program, he did not get any better. Because of his illness, he was now on oxygen. Cody was forced to retire in December 2000. He had worked for the State of Nevada in law enforcement. Nevertheless, because of his job, he could not work with an oxygen tank. They are considered a bomb. He was outraged and depressed when he retired. He felt they could have transferred him to a different job, where his oxygen tanks would not have been a problem. However, that did not happen.

Cody developed, or maybe I should say magnified a "why me" attitude when this occurred. He felt he was too young to be retired. He did not have any hobbies, except for car racing, which he could not do anymore, because of this illness. The circle of frustration. Due to his frustrated attitude, he did not realize, or maybe he did not care at the time, that his behavior from the disease was affecting not just him, but everyone around him.

His inability to move past the traumatic event of retirement got old after a while with the family. He had somewhat disliked his job, but now all of a sudden it was his whole life. He could not see that maybe this was a chance to do something else that he might enjoy. All I felted he had learned from this event was to wallow in self-pity.

Do not get me wrong, change is hard, especially, when you have lost control and have no say. Cody was scared, plus no one wants to face the fact he or she could die. I am not sure how I would have handled the situation if the circumstances were reversed.

During the next few years, Cody's personality changed even more. He used to be fun to be around; now he was angry all the time. As I had said, this was a man who has to be in control of his life at all times. Now he had no control over anything, or whatever was wrong with him. The worst part of this, nothing was working for him, and he was not getting better.

When I was at work, all he did was sit around feeling sorry for himself. He could not or would not quit smoking. Worst yet, he would lie about it. Like you can not smell cigarette smoke? His only exercise was pushing the TV remote and drinking beer. Poor me... Poor me. I am an extrovert and probably a pain in the butt, and with him in this withdrawal behavior, needless to say, it created conflict. Life was in major turmoil for us.

When we would go out, it angered him that he had to pack the oxygen tank. My husband is a shy man and somewhat judgmental, so he didn't like the attention he felt the oxygen tanks drew to him. Being shy, he was usually quiet and retiring, except now he has a terrible temper. Cody became so furious and frustrated that we stopped seeing friends. He had to control all situations, if we were out to dinner or camping, it had to be his way. In talking with a counselor, this is typical behavior for this type of disease. However, it is hell to live with, the flight syndrome comes to mind.

Based on his personality changes, he felted he had to quit things he enjoyed. If he did not want to do it, no one else got to do it either. If I did, there was hell to pay for leaving him home alone. He would sulk and not talk to you. I swear it was like raising another child.

So he had to give up car racing, but there is more to life than racing. You can still attend the races. However, he really did not want to do that either. After much augment, he would occasionally attend, but, hated packing his oxygen.

We participated a little in some hot rod car shows as we still had the 1968 R/T Charger, but not as much. Cars at that time did not bring much joy to him, mainly because he hated people to see him on oxygen. So on many occasions, he would go without the oxygen. This, in turn, due to the lack of oxygen, would make him angrier and moodier. I was glad I was working a sixty-plus-hour job, and the kids were grown up... As it gave me freedom from the chaos at home.

But I have to say, Cody is not a quitter. We were involved with a car event and had been for years. People depended on us to work at this event. He worked his butt off packing his tanks and wearing his mask. It was a four-day event, it about killed him, but he did it. The best part was he did have fun. He may have bitched, but he did enjoy seeing the cars.

I continued to work until 2002, by then Cody was completely on hundred percent oxygen, he had to use tanks when we went out and used a concentrator at home. I could have worked longer but decided to retire to take care of him. At that time, he was on a little over 2 liters of oxygen, which is not bad, but he needed someone around to keep an eye on him. The lack of oxygen also affects the mind in remembering things. Therefore, he had a bit of temporary dementia.

Let me explain how oxygen works and what it means. The human body requires at least 90% oxygen to keep functioning correctly. When the body drops below 90% your heart, lungs, and brain work harder because they are deprived of air. Due to the lack of proper levels of oxygen, it affects the personality. In Cody case, he just became extremely frustrated and angry.

+++

We had been going to Reno to the Doctors for almost two years. These Doctors were specialized in lung diseases or at least, was supposed to, but I had my doubts. I sometimes wonder how many people died because of their incompetence, but I am getting ahead of myself with the story.

Cody started carrying an oximeter to check his oxygen levels. (The attending pulmonary physicians never told us about this piece of equipment. We had to learn about it from friends and on the Internet.) So basically, to keep Cody at 90% we had to add almost two more liters of oxygen with each breath he took, so he was now up to over four liters.

Over those years, not months, but years. Cody kept getting worst. Medical care in Nevada has improved since then, but not by much, I am sorry to say. The group of pulmonary Doctor's we saw in Reno did not seem to care or notice how bad he was getting over this length of time. Each time we had an appointment; we had a different doctor. We would go through the whole history with each Doctor, as it seems they never read his medical file before the visit. Then that Doctor would send him for the same test as the Doctor before him. It was frustrating for both of us. However, thank goodness, his oxygen level through all this was staying around four liters.

But our troubles kept building up. The co-pay costs for the oxygen were starting to add up, so we went to the Veteran's Administration seeing Cody was a retired Major from the Air Force. We were denied benefits based on the fact I made too much money. If Cody had gotten out of the service during the Vietnam era, they would have covered him. However, he retired out after the Cold War, and his benefits were then calculated by our income. Seeing, I made too much money, this disqualified him from receiving any benefits. I told them we were not married when this accident occurred in the missile silo, but they did not care.

We went to our Senator's office and requested assistances in this matter; he got us an appeal. Again, we were denied. The Regional Director told us if I divorced him, they would cover his medical. I could not believe this. This was a man who dedicated a portion of his life to keeping America safe.

I informed the Director, which way the sun shined... It did not get Cody any help, but it made me feel better. I picked up a part-time job to help with the medical cost. Thank gosh, we had good insurance, even so, the co-pays were killing us. All those tests requested by the Doctors plus the oxygen have co-pays.

Cody became harder and harder to live with, he didn't trust the Doctors, and I couldn't blame him. It seems everything was against him. The Doctors had diagnosed him with COPD, Lung Cancer and finally said, we do not know what is wrong with him, but again, I am getting ahead of myself with the story.

+++

We are a close, supportive family, but everyone walked on eggshells when they came to visit. He became even more cynical and frustrated. He was so incredibly upset that the littlest thing would start him off. Then he would throw things and cuss like a sailor. He was hell to be around, so everyone started staying away. If I had been a weaker person and did not have a great support group, I would have left him – the flight emotion again.

I could not do anything right, if fact, none of the family could. He complained about everyone and everything because he had lost control and was so ill. His oxygen levels, thank goodness, were still around four to five liters on the concentrator.

Then in 2005, life changed even more for us.

Chapter Two - The Accident

Mid-January 2005, things started a downhill slide. We had a cold, wet winter with lots of snow and ice. While taking the dogs out, Cody slipped and fell on the ice and shattered his wrist, he had to have four pins put in. Now he had a wrist in a cast and packing his oxygen bottles when we went out, all this just added to his pleasant personality.

When we were home, he was still sitting on the couch, smoking while breathing through a plastic tube from the concentrator or on his computer. Either way, we were all miserable. Cody preferred to be by himself. He spent a lot of time in the bedroom watching TV. If he were on the couch in the front room, then I would disappear. We did not talk much as neither one of us were happy.

However, before the accident, Cody had become a travel agent, working at home. Thank goodness, gave him something to do, beside bitch. He had planned for us to go on an eight-day cruise to Mexico in early February. After the accident, I said, let's cancel, but Cody insisted we go. It was going to be too hard on both of us, but I think he thought this might be his last vacation. It was going to be interesting for both of us getting around. Him packing an oxygen tank with a cast and me with my bad knees.

Before the cruise, we had to fly to the ship in Los Angeles. This was an experience all of its own. At the airport going through security check, seeing he was on oxygen, security took his e-tank away from him to check to see if it was a bomb. They had it so long, he started turning blue from lack of oxygen. I called it "Smurfing" for the little blue people in the children's cartoon.

I had to tell security; "You are killing my husband over there." Pointing to my husband. The security agent could see he was in stress. People do not understand oxygen use. They think it is only used to cure a hangover or a matter of choice to be on it.

As I explained to the security officer. "To understand what it is like for people needing oxygen close your mouth, press closes one nostril and press on the other nostril off and on. You can't get enough air".

After my explanation, he understood and gave Cody back his tank. Like they could have x-rayed it anyway. I do marvel at the stupidity of people.

Millions of people use oxygen. However, there are still people who just do not understand what it is like to be short of air. Also, I found that people are very judgmental, "Oh, you smoked." like you deserve being on oxygen. People can beat their children, wife, but God forbid do not smoke!

Thank gosh, Cody ordered oxygen to be aboard the ship when we arrived, he would have E-tanks and a concentrator. That was a blessing as we couldn't have packed enough air for eight days. I knew I would have to pack most everything else, which was okay. I kept it to two suitcases. The good thing about the trip, besides the warm weather, was I found a way to leave him occasionally and unbelievably he did have fun.

Needless to say, the trip to Mexico was a challenge. If you have ever been on a cruise, it is a problem getting on the ship all by themselves, let alone with a handicap; it was interesting, but we made it.

Once on the Island Princess, things went well. We had a fantastic room; we could hear the quiet whoosh of the vessel moving through the water from the balcony, the wind in your ears, and the ships' flags flapping in the wind. Also, we could sunbathe on the balcony with the concentrator in the cabin, so it worked out well. I love the sounds of the accented voices of ship employees, and they take such good care of you.

The warm weather was a change from all the snow we had left at home. The food on the Cruise was excellent. I love all the different types of food on the menu and on the ship, plus you could eat in your room. Cody had a great time and enjoyed the evening shows. Maybe this cruise was good for both of us. The best part was he took his oxygen with him, as he felt no one knew him and he saw other men using oxygen.

We took a bus ride into Mazatlan, a Nahuatl word meaning "place of the deer," is within ten miles of the Pacific coast. Mazatlan is also right below the Tropic of Cancer, which puts it at the same latitude as Honolulu. Because of its location, Mazatlan had very mild weather and little rain. Throughout the year, temperatures generally range from 68 to 75 degrees Fahrenheit.

Mazatlan is also known as the "Pearl of the Pacific," and is Mexico's largest commercial port. In fact, Mazatlan is one the major West Coast seaports, behind only the Los Angeles port, and the Panama Canal. Because of the port's size, it is a stop for many cruises.

The harbor in Mazatlan is the meeting point for the Sea of Cortez and the Pacific Ocean. This creates one of the greatest natural fish traps in the world, which explains why sport fishing is one of Mazatlan's favorite pastimes.

Due to its location, it is no small wonder that Mazatlan houses the Mexico's largest shrimp fleet, one of Mexico's largest tuna fleets, and the biggest tuna canning factories on the Pacific coast. We got to see all of these sights and eat the food.

The city of Mazatlan is filled with plenty to do. There are many family oriented activities, as well as great places to visit around the city, such as the Aquarium and Mazatlan's beautiful beaches. We visited the Pacifico brewery, which is one of the country's largest breweries. We enjoyed our four-hour tour of Mazatlan.

Our next stop was Puerto Vallarta. We hired a small van for six people and a guide to see the sights. He took us to see where John Huston's 1964 film, "The Night of the Iguana" was filmed and told us all about how it was filmed. Liz Taylor came to keep an eye on her lover Richard Burton while he was filming with the voluptuous Ava Gardner. The publicity buzz about Burton and Liz's torrid affair and the movie put Vallarta on the tourist map.

Otherwise, Puerto Vallarta, a just sleepy fishing village on the Pacific Coast, where the states of Jalisco and Nayarit meet. The Puerto Vallarta region is actually several destinations rolled into one, each with its own character and charm. The River Cuale divides the town into north and south. At the southern end is the quaint Romantic Zone, where the Playa Los Muertos attracts sun worshippers to its golden sand and many beach bars.

Further south the seaside villages of Boca de Tomatlan and Mismaloya, where "The Night of the Iguana" was filmed. North of the river, the Old Town meanders uphill to Gringo Gulch and along the bay where you'll find the Plaza de Armas (main square) and Los Arcos amphitheater where daily free performances draw crowds.

Puerto Vallarta's renowned Malecón (seaside promenade) runs from the Romantic Zone to the start of the Hotel Zone. Here you'll find a whimsical collection of bronze sculptures, including the town's iconic seahorse. Further north is the Hotel Zone and Marina where many resorts and restaurants are located. The locals seem genuinely happy to welcome us. You may be encouraged to practice your Spanish, but pretty much everyone speaks English. The hot, humid, rainy season lasts from June to October, which we missed in February. However, the weather was great and in the 80's.

Once you get away from the beach, Puerto Vallarta's hilly cobblestone streets seem to merge into the green foothills of the Sierra Madre Mountains. We doubt they sell many Stair Masters here; we got our exercise just navigating up, and around town, it about killed us. Oh well, we slept well at night.

Along with golden beaches, mountains and jungles we discovered modern amenities and creature comforts. In short, Puerto Vallarta is a very simpatico and affordable paradise that appeals to everyone. Our highlight of the stop was we went to a tequila factory and watched how they made the liquor the old fashion way. It tastes pretty darn good too, had to buy a few bottles to bring home.

The last stop that we sailed into, Cabo San Lucas.

Again, we took a bus tour of Cabo San Lucas (Spanish pronunciation: [ˈkaβo san ˈlukas], Cape Saint Luke), commonly called Cabo in American English, is a city at the southern tip of the Baja California Peninsula and almost everyone speaks English.

Cabo has been rated as one of Mexico's top five tourist destinations; it is known for its beaches, scuba diving locations, the sea arch El Arco de Cabo San Lucas, and marine life.

Cabo houses a range of wildlife, including rays, sharks, birds like eagles and different types of fish like mahi-mahi and stripe marlin. I did a little snorkeling in the bay. We also took a boat tour to see where the two seas meet, the Pacific Ocean and the Gulf of California. We visited Cabo Wabo Cantina and drank beer at the Baja Brewing Company. It was a great vacation.

+++

When we came home from Mexico, Cody started feeling bad. He would not go to a Doctor. We raise his oxygen level to six liters, thinking that would help. It did not.

He would say "why should I go to the Doctors, they don't know what is wrong with me and they don't care."

The sad part Cody was right, they didn't care, they would just have him take the same tests for the insurance money. Not feeling well, Cody was limited in what he could do, if he walked from the front room to the kitchen, he was out of breath, and his stats would drop below 90%. He still would not go to the Doctor.

At the end of February a few weeks after we came home from the cruise. He had the pins removed from his wrist at the orthopedic office, and I told the Doctor about what was going on with Cody. The Doctor checked him out, Cody's SATS (oxygen levels) were at that time at 77%, remember he needed to be at 90%; the Doctor said this was not his field, but things were not right. At that moment, he had his nurse physically wheel Cody to the hospital. Thank goodness, their office was across the street from the hospital. God bless his actions.

In ER, they gave him steroids to open up his airways and to get the stats up. Then he went to a hospital in Reno by ambulance. He was in the hospital for ten days. They placed him in isolation due to the fact he had been in Mexico, thinking, maybe he had picked up a virus. This meant the Doctors, Nurses, and visitors had to suit up in paper suits to take care of him or to see him.

Our wonderful Pulmonary Doctors and I say Doctors as every day it was a different Doctor. They proceeded to diagnose him with everything from pneumonia to lung cancer. It was a circus. Talk about an emotional roller coaster. They ran all kinds of tests. They did not have a clue as to what was wrong with him.

As a last resort, they did a bronchoscopy, and everything came back okay.

"A Bronchoscopy is a procedure which an examiner uses a viewing tube to evaluate a patient's lung and airways, including the voice box and vocal cord, trachea, and many branches of bronchi. A Pulmonologist or a thoracic surgeon usually performs a bronchoscopy. Although a bronchoscope does not allow for direct viewing and inspection of the lung tissue itself, samples of the lung tissue can be biopsied through the bronchoscope for examination in the laboratory."

The sample grows in a petri dish to see what infection he might have contacted. Finally, they sent him home without ever finding out what was wrong with him, all of this costing us thousands of dollars. Thank goodness, the steroids helped get his stat level where it belonged, and he was maintaining on four liters of oxygen.

All of this indecisive diagnosis created more frustration and anger in both the family and us. We have a team of pulmonary Doctors who did not know what is wrong with him and really did not care. What is a person to do?

+++

Everything I read, I knew COPD wouldn't cause what

was happening to him. As I stated earlier, we never got the same doctor. So on our next visit; I pitched a fit about this. Finally, after two years, they assigned one Doctor to us. She again ran all kinds of tests. Basically, what they had already done at the hospital, more co-pays to pay. They found nothing new. This was March 2005, the Doctor said, "We will see Cody in six months, stay on the inhalers and that was it!!"

Things did not improve, he was stable on the air at four liters, but he had no ambition. He would tire quickly. We spent most of the summer staying close to home.

After the six months, during the September visit, the Doctor told us, "I don't know what his problem is. We have been treating him for COPD, but nothing is working." She further stated, "All the tests came back okay."

I thank her for her honesty, but as his wife; it was something I did not want to hear. "Something is wrong with him, and maybe it is not COPD." I further said to the Doctor, "If you don't know, then refer him to someone or somewhere who can find out what is wrong."

She never did, nor did the Doctors' office...

+++

Shortly after this frustrating visit, we contacted Cody's primary Doctor, who had admitted earlier he had no experience in this field, but he would get a referral for us. He requested to have Cody sent to Stanford in California. The insurance company, however, would not approve Stanford. They did, though approve sending Cody to the National Jewish Hospital in Denver, Colorado. This was a godsend and the start of a whole new thought process

Chapter Three – The Start of our Journey

We had an appointment for the middle of December 2005 for tests by the National Jewish Hospital. We flew to Denver on United Airlines TED as they could set up oxygen for Cody on the plane, for a cost. He was a little over four liters; however, the plane could only do four liters. We made it do, giving him five liters before the trip and after to keep his stats up.

We make it through security in a wheelchair and with the Doctors order; they did not take his e-tanks from him. He could not walk the distances of the airports, in either Reno or Denver. So thank goodness for the wheelchair.

Cody was born in Denver, he was the youngest of three children. His brother is ten years older, and his sister is five years older, so he was like an only child. We were blessed that his sister Mary and brother-in-law, Bob still live in the area. They picked us up at the airport, and we spent the week with them. This saves us on the cost of a motel and a car. Money was getting tight.

Bob drove us to the National Jewish Hospital every day. We had to spend the whole day there, going for five days. Cody was tested for four days, and I received training to understand his illness and the effects on the family. Poor Bob had to spend all that time in Denver; he said he did not mind, thank goodness for family. I knew a lot of the information, but I learned many new things too. They taught me about his diet; some food upset the lungs more than others, and about all the different types of oxygen. It was all interesting and helpful. The counseling was the best, teaching me how to cope with his personality changes now and later.

"The different types of oxygen a patient may have are the following:

Stationary systems provide a large source of oxygen. However, they restrict movement. The most common and most economical in-home stationary system used is an oxygen concentrator. Concentrators use an electric motor. They work by removing nitrogen from room air to make 94-98 percent oxygen.

A concentrator needs an electrical source. It operates by passing room air through a powder or a membrane to separate oxygen from nitrogen. The oxygen is concentrated and delivered. The nitrogen is regularly released back into the air. Concentrators can be relatively small, weighing anywhere from 22-70 pounds. They can provide a liter flow rate of up to five to six liters per minute. A long supply tubing of about 50 feet in length is needed. This will allow for moving around the house and preventing tangles with furniture.

Since electricity is required, you will also want to have a backup oxygen supply in case of a power failure. And your health care provider should let your electric company know about your oxygen needs. (Note: In Southern California, the electric companies require the customer, not the home care provider, to notify the power company.)

These units must be placed in an open, ventilated area. They must be kept away from heat and flames. Concentrators need routine maintenance. They need inspections, filter changes, and oxygen analysis. Some of the newer models provide an oxygen concentration gauge. This measures the oxygen level delivered by the concentrator. It sounds an alarm if the reading falls below a certain level.

Another stationary system is a reservoir of liquid oxygen. Liquid oxygen is gas condensed into a liquid state by extreme cold. Liquid systems have a large reservoir tank. This tank is filled by the oxygen supplier once or twice a month. These systems require no electricity. They have very few moving parts. They require little maintenance or repair. When dealing with liquid oxygen, caution must be exercised to prevent spills. Liquid oxygen is very cold. It can injure the skin instantly upon contact.

A typical liquid oxygen reservoir weighs 124 pounds when filled. It contains 31 liters, or 73 pounds, of liquid. This amount of liquid oxygen is the same as 24,950 liters of oxygen in the gas form. At a flow rate of two liters per minute, this amount of oxygen would last 208 hours or eight days. Liquid systems consistently lose oxygen through evaporation, even when not in use. So they are suitable for regular use at home, or for filling up portable units. They are not suitable as an emergency backup system. Newer units are now available that reduce the amount of oxygen lost into the air. These new systems also have improvements in size and stability. Many of these systems have built-in pulsed delivery or conserving devices.

Compressed gas oxygen in large tanks or cylinders, commonly known as E-tanks is another example of a stationary system. The Large steel or aluminum tanks are heavy. They cannot be moved easily. They must be safely secured to prevent them from falling over. They are not appropriate for someone who requires continuous flow oxygen. This is because of the volume required to meet a continuous need and the high cost. **(Info from National Jewish)**

Many months later, Cody was packing E-tanks in a metal container, which held four tanks, they only lasted him about twenty minutes...

+++

On the fifth day at National Jewish, the Doctor, after reviewing all the tests, gave us the results. We did not know what to expect after all we had been through, with the other Doctors. He proceeded to tell us, Cody did have COPD; however, it was only a small spot in one lung, that wasn't what was causing his health problem.

The Doctor wasn't exactly sure what was wrong. He said it could be emphysema, asthma, or Intra-Statal Disease, but he knew it was a lot more than COPD.

I asked, "Is it lung cancer?"

He said, "no way. It was not lung cancer."

The Doctor then prescribed some medications, which he hoped would control the problem. He further stated we should know within thirty days if this is working. I thought *not thirty months, but thirty days, what a relief. We may finally find out what is wrong with Cody.*

The Doctor expressed his disappointment with the Doctors in Nevada, as you know; this is unusual for another Doctor to do. However, that is how badly they had misdiagnosed and their lack of treatment for my husband's illness. We did not intend to sue the Doctors in Nevada, and we let the issue drop. The main thing was getting Cody well.

At this time, Cody was on five liters of oxygen. He was to take the prescribed medication for 90 days. Then would have his blood work done monthly and come back to Denver in March for additional testing. The Doctor felt this medicine would help and maybe turn things around. We were so excited that somebody had found something wrong beside COPD and better yet, they were trying to do something about it.

Back home, after thirty days, Cody had his blood work drawn. A few days after the blood work was sent to Denver, National Jewish Hospital called asking to see Cody right away. At this time, however, Cody could no longer fly as he was on six+ liters of oxygen. The oxygen level had increased over the thirty days, as he was getting worst. They told us to get there as soon as we could.

To make this jaunt, we had to have our Motorhome equipped with an electrical inverter. That way we could run the oxygen concentrator while we were driving the sixteen-hour trip. We knew we could not pack enough oxygen tanks for the journey to Denver. We would have had to pack twenty oxygen tanks plus a concentrator to make the journey. Our RV would have been a bomb if we had an accident. Because of having this electrical procedure put in the RV, we could not leave right away.

Ten days later, we were driving to Denver; it took us three days to get there. We had to stop at RV parks each evening to charge the batteries on the inverter. Seeing it was also winter, we also had to take the southern route to Denver through Arizona and New Mexico, which is longer. We arrived in Denver the latter part of February 2006.

The Doctors at National Jewish Hospital ran tests for three more days. On the fourth day, the Doctor called us in and showed slides of everything going on in Cody's lungs. He was very thorough in his explaining of what was going on as we had many questions.

The conclusion of the several Doctors was that Cody needed a double lung and heart transplant. He needed it as soon as possible due to pulmonary hypertension and other complications. The natural history of various interstitial diseases varies. Idiopathic pulmonary fibrosis, of the usual interstitial variant (UIP), which is the second most frequent disease for which lung transplantation is performed, has a median survival of approximately 2.5 to 3.5 years from the time of diagnosis. Seeing we were misdiagnosed, we had lost valuable time. Because of the dismal survival rates for Cody, he was placed on a waiting list indicating that he would receive an early referral for the transplantation process.

The Doctor warned us that we did not have much time left because they caught the disease so late. They gave us, maybe six months to receive his lungs. All of this information and the time restraints were overwhelming. We both cried. We were happy and angry all at the same time. If the Doctors in Reno had correctly diagnosed him, we would have had more time. Some people have to wait for years to get their lungs, and we did not have that kind of time. However, we were thankful as he still had some time left to get this fixed or at least, we hoped. The reality of it all is we were numb and not sure what was going to happen. Cody and I were angry as no one wants to face death when it could have or should have been avoided.

+++

Before we had gone back to Denver on this requested trip, I had spent hours doing research on the computer. We thought that they might do a lung reduction surgery; we never expected they would recommend a double lung and heart transplant. Below explains the different procedures for one type of lung surgery:

"**A Lung Volume Reduction Surgery** (LVRS) is a procedure to help people with severe emphysema. LVRS is not a cure for emphysema, but can improve one's quality of life and can be an alternative to lung transplantation. The goal of the surgery is to reduce the size of the lungs by removing about 30% of the most diseased lung tissues so that the remaining healthier portion can perform better. LVRS can also allow the diaphragm to return to its normal shape, allowing the patient to breathe more efficiently. The surgery has been shown to help improve breathing ability, lung capacity, and overall quality of life." (***National Jewish site***)

National Jewish Hospital is only a diagnostic hospital, and they do not do surgery. Therefore, they referred Cody to Colorado University. I researched the University, and they had one of the highest rates for a double lung surgery, at a 60% success. That made us feel better, even though we were scared. I was petrified but had to show a strong front to Cody and vice versa. We both were numb and just put one foot in front of the other, not really thinking about the negative. Plus, thnk goodness, Cody is a fighter.

The initial lung transplantation program at The University of Colorado was initiated in 1991, and the first lung transplant took place in February 1992. Since its inception, the lung transplant team at The University of Colorado has performed over 450 transplants. They are rated in the top ten hospitals for this type of surgery.

After more tests by the Pulmonary Doctors at the University, it is now the first part of March 2006. They placed Cody on the waiting transplant list for double lungs. The lung transplant team evaluates each referral in view of potential risks and benefits to the patient and the ability and experience of the individuals at the transplant center. The following are some of the issues related to contraindications:

Age

Ventilator dependence

Corticosteroid therapy

Psychosocial issues

Infection

Body weight

Extrapulmonary organ dysfunction

The Doctors at the University (CU), said we did not have enough time to get lungs and a heart, so they were going to try and receive the double lungs only. All of this has been just overwhelming. This type of surgery was a major game changer for everyone. Tons of questions and thoughts go through your mind.

"Note: Information about Lungs Transplants.

Lung transplants are given to people as a last resort treatment for irreversible lung failure. Lung failure happens when the lungs are damaged and unable to transfer oxygen and carbon dioxide to and away from cells. Some diseases that cause the lungs to fail and are treated with transplants are emphysema, including the form caused by the alpha-1-antitrypsin-deficiency, pulmonary fibrosis, cystic fibrosis, and pulmonary hypertension.

In 2005, approximately 3,500 people in the U.S. were waiting for a lung transplant, yet only 1,000 of them (25 percent) received a transplant. Unfortunately, with the improvement of surgical techniques and the expansion of reasons for transplants, the number of needed lung transplants has not kept pace with the number of available donors. To learn more about becoming an organ donor, visit www.organdonor.gov." (Info from CU)

Making the decision about whether to get a lung transplant when it involves life and death of your loved one may seem easy, but getting the transplant has more risks than any other major operation. There may be surgical complications such as major bleeding, pneumonia and pulmonary edema and possibly painful recovery. Also, Cody will have the burden of taking medication that lowers his immune system response and exposes him to lots of serious side effects, including cancer, for the rest of his life.

Also, we will receive counseling to see if he could mentally accept a gift from a donor and handle the responsibility of a transplant. They also wanted to make sure I could accept the concept. It is quite a process for everyone involved. No one makes this choice lightly. The University put both of us through and intensive training to understand the transplant process. They want to ensure we understood what was going to happen before and the after effects.

More information on transplants: "Transplant recipients also have a high risk of rejection and infection. Since the transplanted lungs are considered foreign to the body, there is a risk that the body's immune system will attack and reject the new transplant. Doctors prescribe immunosuppressive (anti-rejection) medication, which lowers immunity to prevent rejection but also increases the risk of infection and other diseases. Rejection most often occurs in the first three months after transplantation, but medication may need to be taken indefinitely.

A team of specially trained staff (pulmonologists, surgeons, immunologists' social workers, nurses, and technicians) evaluates patients to establish whether he or she would be a good candidate for a lung transplant. The person's physical and psychological health and suitability for major surgery are taken into account.

When the Doctors consider a patient to be a good candidate, their name is placed on a national waiting list for an organ transplant. Waiting time may extend several years. Unfortunately, the majority of qualified candidates will not live longer than 1 or 2 years without a transplant. In 2004, close to 533 people waiting for a lung transplant died.

Once there is a deceased lung donor, a ranked list of people is computer-generated. The transplant recipient is chosen based on certain requirements, including immune markers that match the donor, lung size, length of time on the waiting list and proximity to the donor. Each transplant center may have additional criteria also. Once a candidate is chosen, time is critical. The lung must be transplanted into the patient receiving the organ within four to six hours.

Depending on the chosen recipients' need, a single or double lung transplant may be performed. Double lung transplants involve an incision below the breasts and take about 6-12 hours of surgery. For single lung transplants, the incision is made on the side of the body where the lung is to be replaced; the operation takes about 4-8 hours. Once the lungs are replaced, the blood vessels and airway are attached.

In some cases where the heart has been weakened, both the heart and lungs will be replaced. Until 1989, combined heart-lung transplants were the most common form of lung transplantation. Since then, single lung transplants have become the most common form.

After surgery, the patient will make frequent trips to the medical center and have a prescribed home-based rehabilitation program, including physical activity, breathing exercises, nutrition and taking medications especially immunosuppressive drugs. Walking is recommended to restore strength and prevent lung complications. An activity that is more strenuous can resume when one is comfortable. Current survival rates are as high as 80 percent at one year following transplantation and 60 percent at four years.

Lungs can also be transplanted from living donors, adding to the supply of available organs. A living lung donor can be anyone who matches the recipient, related or not. At least two other people have to donate lobes to form an entire lung for one recipient; lobes of the lung are donated depending on which sections of the lungs need to be replaced. Living lung transplants are advantageous because recipients do not have to wait on a list and the transplant can be scheduled at a time convenient for both parties. Also, the recipient can begin to take immunosuppressive medication earlier, which decreases the chances of rejection. Living lung transplants tend to be more successful also because there is a closer match between the donor and recipient. Unfortunately, as of now, the living donor program for lungs is in its infancy, so it will not be available for most people needing a transplant at this time.

For more information about issues related to lung transplants, contact your local American Lung Association at 1-800-LUNG-USA (1-800-586-4872). "

Survival: According to the registry of the International Society for Heart and Lung Transplantation, 1-year, 3-year, and 5-year actuarial survival after lung transplantation are 70.7, 54.8, and 42.6 %, respectively, with a median survival of 3.7 years. Survival rates for lung transplantation have improved only moderately over the past decade, despite refinements in surgical technique and postoperative care. These rates lag considerably behind those for heart and liver transplantation, for which five-year survival is approximate 70%.

The death rate is highest in the year after transplantation, with infection and graft failure representing the leading causes of early death. Factors that portend a poorer prognosis include a pre-transplantation diagnosis of pulmonary hypertension, dependence on a ventilator, and age of more than 50 in the recipient or donor.

I placed all of this information throughout the story for people to understand the transplant process. It is a very emotional choice as you cannot pray for some to die to receive the lungs, yet you are praying for a family member to stay alive long enough to receive them. This is a very dangerous surgery medically and emotionally.

Cody was on every prayer list I could find. As I sat in Doctor's office, I would talk to total strangers to have them pray for him. I did not care what faith they practiced; just keep him in your prayers.

Chapter Four   Living in Denver

We thought about going back home to Nevada. But after further consideration, we thought it would be better to wait in Denver, closer to the hospital. Patients who are accepted as potential transplant candidates must carry a pager with them at all times in case a donor organ becomes available. Cody must also be prepared to move to their chosen transplant center at a moment's notice. Cody was encouraged to limit our travel and stay within a certain geographical region in order to facilitate rapid transport to a transplant center. Therefore, we stayed in the Denver area.

Moreover, Cody was getting worse; he was now on twelve to fifteen liters of oxygen. Therefore, if he could not fly, we would not meet the four to six-hour window to be at the hospital for the surgery. So there was no going back to Nevada. We looked into the Fisher House, seeing Cody is a veteran, he would qualify. However, they did not allow pets. We had brought our two small dogs and two cats with us.

We look around the Denver area and found an RV park. They aren't many Recreation Vehicle (RV) parks in the area. We ended up staying at an RV Park in Wheatridge. We were lucky as they had room for our RV. Wheatridge is a rural community about fifteen miles from Denver, so we could make it to the hospital in a timely manner. I loved the park, as it felt like home, I so dislike big cities. As it turned out, we stayed in the Park for almost a year.

The RV Park proved to be another blessing, as the owners of the Park became like family. They were so supportive over the next few months, as so were many other people staying at the park. I met Millie and her dogs and Joe, a physical education teacher, running away from life. I felt like I was at home in Nevada. I grew up in Nevada and had only left a couple of times to go to school. I consider myself a country-bumpkin, so Wheatridge fits me just fine. Cody sister only lived about thirty miles away, so it was a perfect spot.

Within, a hundred miles radius of Denver there are three million people. In Nevada, we barely have over two million inhabitants in the whole state. The only City in Nevada that compares to Denver is Las Vegas, which is seven hours from where we live. We live on a two-lane road in rural Nevada. So driving to the hospital on a six-lane freeway was a challenge, especially at peak times. People drive 60-70 mph bumper to bumper!! And never use their blinkers. Also, in Colorado, you do not stop for emergency vehicles, I did stop once because, in Nevada, it is the law. However, in Colorado I got tooted, cuss at and shown I was number one. It was a learning experience. I just learned I hated big cities...

While we waited for the lungs, Cody had to go to the hospital in Denver twice a week for physical therapy. Which about killed him as he was so weak. He is now on fifteen liters of oxygen. Cody's drive was something else, I have to commend him, and he never gave up. Cody's will-to-live was unbreakable. He had a goal to survive so he could receive the surgery.

They placed Cody on the transplant list the first part of March 2006 for double lungs. We were not on the top, but close. As stated, he needed double lungs and a heart, but we did not have enough time to receive them all.

"When your transplant center has identified you as an eligible candidate for a lung transplant, the Northeast Ohio Organ Procurement Agency (known as LifeBanc) enters your name and blood type on the United Network for Organ Sharing's (UNOS) computerized national waiting list. This waiting list assures equal access and fair distribution of organs when they become available.

When a lung becomes available for transplantation, it is given to the best possible match, based on blood type, size, tissue (HLA) type, recipient's medical condition, crossmatch compatibility, the length of time the recipient has been waiting, and the number of lungs the recipient needs." (CU procedures)

Cody's level of oxygen needs kept going up, by the time of the surgery, he was on twenty-seven liters. In fact, the hospital only went to twenty-five liters. Cody's amount of air was unheard of, the hospital could not believe him and his will to live. He should have been dead before the surgery.

We had two fifteen-liter concentrators in the RV. He

couldn't walk from the bedroom to the kitchen in the thirty-foot motor home, without being out of breath. It would take him forever, just to take a shower. When we went out, He would go through four E-tanks in twenty minutes. This was enough air to get him to the hospital to do his exercise, and then he would hook up four more tanks to get him into the hospital. He would need four tanks to get to the car, then four more to get back to the RV. Figuring that out; that is sixteen tanks for each trip twice a week. We would get forty tanks a week equaling hundred and sixty a month. The cost of the air was only covered 50% by the insurance; the rest of the cost was ours.

His personality may have had the drive to live during this process, but he was hell to live with. I threaten a few times; I was going to kink his oxygen hose. If we were not going to the hospital, we stayed in the RV. The stress from all of this was overwhelming.

The Park had a laundry, so once a week I got away from the RV and talked with other people. My other chore was cleaning the RV around all the air hoses. Life was interesting, but we survived.

When the weather got warm, I planted a little garden in pots and bought some flowers to bloom outside the rig. We tried to make the coach as comfortable as possible... home away from home.

My only link to home and family was through e-mail and phone. I have enclosed the emails, which will appear later in this story, as I wrote to family and friends every day he was in the hospital.

Chapter Five – The First Call

The end of March we got a call for the double lung surgery. We couldn't believe our luck, so soon. We called everybody as we were so excited. He was going to make it, and all would be okay. Life was good.

The procedure for a transplant, is they call to prepare you so you can make it to the hospital during the limited time frame. They then will give you a final call to confirm the surgery and how much time you have. It is crucial that the Doctor team and you meet that time frame. If too much time lapses, the lungs can go to waste.

As we waited for final confirmation, we were so excited and doing our happy dance. He was going to get his lungs. Then the call came canceling the surgery. We were devastated.

Later, in talking with other recipients waiting for transplants, we found this to be commonplace. One lady had been called six times before she received her lungs. However, with everything we had gone through, all the counseling, no one had warned us about this emotional disappointment. We cried. It was a terribly long night. Cody just got angrier.

We waited some more. Which is quite hard. Cody knew he was dying, but we waited. As stated, he had to go to the hospital two times a week. We would make the drive to the hospital in Denver. Cody had to drive to the hospital, as he would not relinquish control. This trip was hard on Cody. He had to walk about a quarter of a mile to the exercise facilities. As stated, it would take four E-tanks to make this journey. I would then go back to the car and get four new tanks for him to make the trip back to the car. We did this for four-plus months.

Cody and the dogs would walk around the RV Park every day, very slowly, but by damn, he did it, better than I could. There was a beautiful lake beside the park, which we could see from the Motorhome. He wanted to walk there, but it was not going to happen, at least not now. Later he would walk it every day with the dogs.

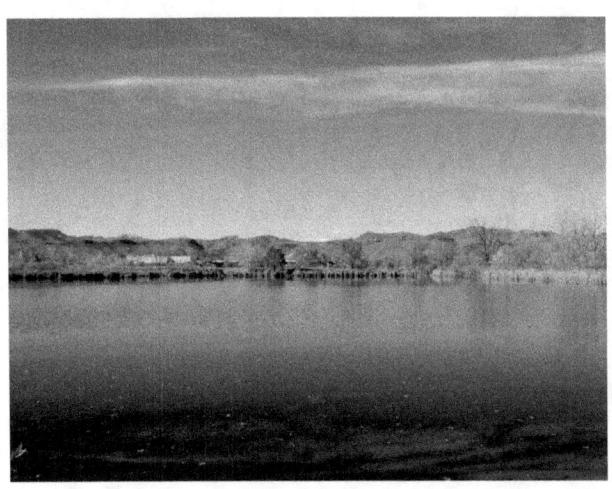

We waited... and we waited... no news. Cody could not

do much except watch TV. We would visit with his sister on Sunday for dinner, but traveling was hard on Cody, they lived about thirty miles from Wheatridge. We would pack about twenty tanks for the trip and take the concentrator.

In April that year, we had snow. We had the awning out on the RV, and it was well braced to handle the snow, if not I would go out with a broom and knock it off. We had a propane man come by twice a month to give us gas, as Cody would get real cold. Plus, we ran electric heaters. The Denver area is higher in humility than Nevada, and we both felt the weather. Cody walked whenever the weather would let him. He was now on eighteen liters of oxygen. We waited for a second call... none.

May came, and the weather was a little warmer. Apparently, Colorado was having a light winter. Cody walked with the dogs but was now on twenty liters of oxygen. We still made our trips to the hospital in Denver to exercise. He would do that until the surgery; if and when we get called. We would go to the store, and once in a while out to dinner at a Mexican restaurant, that was close to the Park. Other than that we stayed close to home and waited... no call came.

June came, and we still waited. We had developed a routine, twice a week trip to the hospital and Sunday dinner with his sister, the rest of time was spent in the RV. Cody was now on the top of the transplant list. He was now on twenty-two to twenty-five liters of oxygen. We were basically held captive to the RV because of the oxygen level. Linacre had brought us two new fifteen liter concentrators last month to keep up with Cody's needs, plus all the tanks. We had so many we stored them under the coach, plus a trunk full in the car.

We would sit at the kitchen table, me drinking coffee and watch a fox in the park; it would come and eat some of the cat's food. The fox would try to catch the Park's farrow cats. We did not let our cats out unless they were on a leash. As the weather got warmer, Cody could sit at the picnic table and enjoy the summer sun, but that was about it. He was bored and angry. He had no hobbies; he would read occasionally, but mainly he just bitched. He could not walk as far in the park due to the increased need for oxygen. Nevertheless, he stilled walk, got to give him credit for that, this man never gave up.

I was getting worried as Cody was now coughing up blood. I talked to the Doctor in June about this, what do I do if he needs help, as there would not be enough time to get him to Denver. They suggested the local hospital in Wheatridge, so we drove around and found it to be prepared. Hoping we never will use it...

We both knew he was on his last legs. Finally, in July, we got the second call. We did not get excited this time, we took the wait and see attitude. I do not think either one of us was up to being disappointed again, so we just did not get excited. We got the second call to go, but I felt it was not going to happen. As we were getting ready to go, a third call came, canceling the procedure. This call tore us up, as the lungs went to waste. See the e-mail below:

Date: Thu, 6 Jul 2006 09:38:58 -0700 (PDT)

We got a call last night, Denver had a set of lungs coming from Nebraska, they gave us the second call, saying it was a go and we started getting ready to go in, then they called the third time and canceled. This was at 4 am. It seems there was not enough time to get the lungs, as the coroner wanted the body at 7 am because the family wanted the family member by noon. Denver couldn't get there in time and do the surgery. OPN (the transplant Org) sat on the lungs too long, I guess the lung was to go to Minnesota, but that didn't work out then they called Denver, but not enough time left. So we wait some more. However, I think it will be soon.

Cody hasn't been doing well, I just hope it is not too much longer, or he may not be able to handle the surgery. His color is gray, and he is so tired.

We cried some more, and we waited, but we felt we were getting close, or least prayed we were.

However, there was no laughter in our household. The animals were the only ones that made us happy. It is not fun when Cody knew he was dying and as the spouse, you are watching your mate die. We prayed and cried. Neither one of us are patience people, and the waiting was so emotional, or maybe it was the not knowing if we would get lungs in time.

Chapter Six - The Final Call

On July 10, 2006, at 8:30 p.m., while we were watching TV, we got the call, and this time they said it was for real. We called everybody telling them this time it was going to happen. We had to be at the hospital at 10:00 p.m. Mary and Bob came over and drove us to the hospital and gave us both support.

We stayed with him in the pre-operating room, as we waited for the team of doctors to arrive with the lungs. The pre-operating room was cold and very sterile, and depressing. We stayed with him for several hours waiting for the team of Doctors with the lungs, it seemed like forever. The procedure was the Doctors at the hospital would start prepping Cody as soon as the plane landed. Basically, he would be ready to go, and when the doctors got the word, he would then be administered the anesthesia. Below is information on how they harvest the lung and transport:

"With the current techniques, the satisfactory graft function can be obtained after an ischemic interval of as long as 6-8 hours. Ischemic injury to the pulmonary vascular endothelium increases permeability and results in pulmonary edema".

"Hypothermic flush perfusion is the method used most commonly for pulmonary preservation in clinical practice. After systemic hepatization of the donor, the pulmonary vasculature is flushed with a cold solution. Commonly used solutions are modified Euro-Collins solution, University of Wisconsin solution, and Perfadex. These are delivered via a large pulmonary artery cannula at a volume of 50-60 mL/kg over 4-5 minutes. Most flush solutions are administered at a temperature of 4°C, while topical cooling is carried out by filling the pleural cavity with an iced crystalloid solution. The harvested lungs are immersed in crystalloid solution, packed in ice, and transported at a temperature of 1-4°C. The infusion and transport are performed during active ventilation and static inflation with O2 respectively. (CU)

Cody finally got into the surgery around 3:00 a.m. Cody was so scared; this was a man who never had surgery, and he had no control over the procedure or anything that was happening. Basically, before this illness, Cody had never been sick. I hated leaving him with the Doctors as my heart was breaking. *What if he does not make it?*

I knew he had a great team of Doctors and he would be okay or at least I wanted to believe that, but it is still hard, and you still worry. The donor's lungs came from Minneapolis. We found out a year later they came from a 20-year-old college student named Nate. Our precious gift from a stranger named Nate. The younger lungs were a blessing for Cody. However, it was sad that such a young man died, I felt for his mother.

"Requirements for potential donors

There are certain requirements for potential lung

donors, due to the needs of the potential recipient. In the case of living donors, this is also, in consideration of how the surgery will affect the donor. Healthy; size match; the donated lung or lungs must be large enough to adequately oxygenate the patient, but small enough to fit within the recipient's chest cavity; age; and blood type".

The donor gave his lungs to us, and three other people received his liver, kidneys, and pancreas, so that day four people's lives changed. We understood that no one received the heart.

After we had left him, we headed for the waiting room. I gaze over the waiting room, seeking a place for us to sit. I saw a coffee table filled with tattered magazines and travel books, cardboard holders with pamphlets, advertisement posters on the walls, and hallway leading to operating rooms. TV's were playing in all four corners of the large room. Finally, we find one group of chairs away from the crowd.

The waiting room was pleasant enough; people were trying to sleep on the floor. There was the scent of get-well flowers, questionable food smells from food trays and body sweat. People were talking in low voices, intercom calling out codes. It was going to be a long night. Sorry to say the chairs even padded are uncomfortable after sitting in them for hours.

Mary, Bob, and I were seated in the waiting room,

waiting. I was so glad they were with me, as the waiting for this type of surgery is the hardest part, or so I thought. I eyed the dark blue door of the waiting room where the doctor would come through, to tell us what had happened with Cody. I have a vivid imagination, as I imagined it as a black hole that sucked away my husband; I was so scared for him and for us.

About an hour into the surgery, unexpectedly, I started to cry and said, "Cody has died." I could not stop crying. About a minute later, which seemed like forever, I said, "he is back with us." His family thought I was nuts. I have a type of ESP that feels things before or in this case while it is happening. My ESP seems only to work with the people I love. We talked about the incident later during another surgery.

After the surgery when Cody was okay, he remembers dying and seeing a red light and hearing his dead Mother telling him to go back. My husband or his family do not believe in this kind of stuff. However, my husband now believes a little.

Hours went by as we waited for news. We watched TV, Drank burnt coffee, and ate bland food from the vending machines. Finally, eating a meal of Hospital food. We would do anything to stay awake. As I waited, I talked to other people waiting for news of their loved ones. Their stories broke my heart, like the little girl whose hands were clenched in a worry knot, worrying about her Daddy. He had been severely burned, and they were not sure he would make it. (I never did find out if he did survive). They had been there for several days, sleeping on the floor. The elderly man, all by himself, with no family or friends, who looked lost and frightened waiting to hear how his wife was doing. She was having heart surgery. I blinked back tears, my problems didn't seem so serious as Cody was getting a life changing surgery and I had a family for support.

It was over a ten-hour surgery. Dr. W. was exhausted when he came through the blue doors, to see us in the waiting room. His face was haggard. He said it was challenging, but Cody was doing okay now and in recovery. They would place Cody in a medical coma for three to five days. The reason for this was that the lungs needed to be accepted by the body by then and they could also drain the fluid from the lungs. When they transport the lungs, they are on ice. After that, he should be on the mend. Doctor W said, "Be patience as it will take a while."

We could not see Cody as of yet, as he was in recovery and would be there for quite a while. We were welcome to see him, but he was out of it. Doctor W. told us to go home, the worst was over; go get some rest, all would be okay. We went in and saw Cody, it was sad, as he was gray and cold.

The nurse said, "That this was normal and he would be

under for probably an hour or two, due to the length of the surgery."

I held his hand, as you could not hug due to the tubes, told him I loved him and would see him in the morning. We left the hospital around 4:30 p.m. as we all had been up for over 24 hours.

When I got home, I took care of the animals, who were so good. They did not have any accidents. I tried to sleep. This was July 11th. I did not go to the hospital that evening, I called the hospital around 8:00 p.m. and they said he was out of recovery and was in the medicated coma, but everything was looking good. I called all the family, walked the dogs, fed everybody, and went back to bed.

The next morning, I drove to the hospital to see him. I am not easily shocked, but wow, I thought he had a lot of tubes in recovery, there was even more now. He had tubes coming out of him from everywhere. He was on a ventilator tube in his throat with nitro. He was on oxygen, a catheter, IV and blood transfusion going all at the same time. He had five tubes for drainage. They had tubes coming out of all of his orifices, plus coming out from the chest cavity by his ribs. His color was gray, he looked like death warmed over.

"A medical ventilator (or simply ventilator in context) is a machine designed to mechanically move breathable air into and out of the lungs, to provide the mechanism of breathing for a patient who is physically unable to breathe, or breathing insufficiently.Ventilators are chiefly used in intensive care medicine, home care, and emergency medicine (as standalone units) and in anesthesia (as a component of an anesthesia machine).

Medical ventilators are sometimes colloquially called "respirators," a term which stems from commonly used devices in the 1950s (particularly the "Bird Respirator"). However, in modern hospital and medical terminology, these machines are never referred to as respirators, and use of "respirator" in this context is now a deprecated anachronism which signals technical unfamiliarity."

Below is the e-mail I sent to the family and friends. I did this every day, so we would have a record and be thankful for what all he went through. I have not corrected the errors as they are as I sent them.

Date: Wed, 12 Jul 2006 14:10:05 -0700 (PDT)

Subject: Cody

Latest update: Wednesday 2:45

Just got home from the hospital after seeing Cody, was there for a couple of hours. He is still in a coma, trying to come out a few times, but would start to move, so they put him back under. Things today are not where they should be, they gave him two pints of blood last night, two pints this morning, and two while

I was there. They cannot find any leakage, either in the drains or by x-rays.

I talked to several Dr's about his guarded condition. The pulmonary hypertension is causing problems - the arteries from the heart to the lungs. His heart is erratic; it would go from 90 to 117 back to 93 to 102, just jumped around like that, so they are trying to stable the heart.

Because of this, the ventilator will not be removed today and a good chance, not tomorrow. This means he stays in the medically induced coma.

In addition, apparently, when they remove the lungs from the donor, they are filled with a saline solution and place on ice. When the lungs are transferred to Cody, they lower his body temperature to accept the cold lungs and Cody is in a study to help remove the saline solution. The patient does not know if the medicine to dry up the fluid is real or a placebo. Dr. Z thinks Cody received the placebo. So his blood is mixing with the water fluids and creating some concerns, so while I was there, they put him on a laysick (spelled wrong) drip, this will make him pee a lot. Dr. Z wants to take this action to dry him out.

They will call me if any negative changes occur, but basically, he was somewhat stable when I left, except for the heart rate.

He looks better than yesterday and is warm to the touch. I took the stupid pictures he wanted, must be a guy thing!

I talked to him, they said he could hear, so told him what was going on. Gave him everyone love and prayers. So we just wait and see. I will call this evening to see how he is progressing.

Thanks again for everyone support. I will try to e-mail you daily with a report until he is out of the woods.

"**A placebo** (/plə'siboʊ/ plə-SEE-boh; Latin placēbō, is a simulated or otherwise medically ineffectual treatment for a disease or other medical condition intended to deceive the recipient. Sometimes patients given a placebo treatment will have a perceived or actual improvement in a medical condition, a phenomenon commonly called the placebo effect or placebo response. The placebo effect consists of several different effects woven together, and the methods of placebo administration may be as important as the administration itself."

Chapter Seven – Now the Healing Process

I now drove into Denver every day while Cody was in the hospital. I would stay three to four hours and then head back to Wheatridge before heavy traffic. The mousetrap as they call it, can be bumper to bumper at fast speeds if you did not get through it by 2 pm. I was driving Cody's car, which is a little compact. If I had wrecked it, there would be hell to pay, so besides hating big city traffic, I worried about his car.

One time going into the hospital, I had two eighteen wheelers on each side of me, a dump truck in the front and a garbage truck behind me all driving 65 mph and I prayed they did not give me a group hug...

Cody was in a medicated coma for over two weeks. They had said when he came out of the coma, he would go to rehabilitation to exercise the lungs. Medicated comas are a little bit funny, as the person is there, but not. Even when he started coming out of it, the lights were on, but nobody was home. He was fed through a tube in his nose, he had a port in his neck, and also an IV is connected to the port that fed him. He was on oxygen at 2 liters.

"Before a coma can be induced, it's critical the proper equipment and medical personnel be available. The procedure is initiated in an intensive-care unit (ICU), where monitoring technology is available to support the airway and ensure that blood pressure, heart rate and oxygen levels in the blood are maintained at normal levels.

The drugs needed to induce a coma — usually propofol or a barbiturate such as pentobarbital or thiopental — are given to a patient by an infusion pump that administers precisely metered doses. These drugs "have a continuum of effects, allowing the anesthesiologist to gradually take the patient from "general anesthesiology into a deep coma.

The length of time a patient is in a medically induced coma is largely dependent on the disease that you are treating. In most cases, a coma is induced for a few days up to two weeks; induced comas longer than a month are exceedingly rare. It is very much dependent on the individual circumstances.

Risks of a medically induced coma

Like most medical procedures, an induced coma carries some risks. One of the consequences that we do know of is an increased risk of infection. Chest infections are especially common since a coma significantly affects the cough reflex, which helps to remove secretions from the lungs.

Barbiturates, too, can diminish the immune response, though there's not a tremendous wealth of data on that. And the preventative, use of antibiotics is not usually recommended due to their association with the development of antibiotic-resistant bacteria, aka "superbugs."

There is also some controversy over the need for

medically induced comas: Some studies have found limited benefits from barbiturate-induced comas, particularly among people over age 40. A 2004 report from the journal Anesthesia concluded that "the potential benefits of barbiturate coma have to be balanced against the risks. These complications need to be considered when an adverse neurological outcome seems likely."

Comas and nightmares

Some patients who have undergone an induced coma report experiencing vivid nightmares and hallucinations. This attribute the effect to the brain's efforts at trying to make sense of perceptions (especially sounds) from the environment.

As an anesthesiologist, I can tell you that there are a lot of interesting perceptions that patients have as they're emerging from anesthesia. It's relatively common for reporting all sorts of perception following sedations, including some very disturbing hallucinations. There are some fairly vivid nightmares, usually as they're emerging from sedation."

Despite the risks associated with a medically induced coma, the procedure has improved considerably in recent years, mainly due to the advances in monitoring technology; much of the monitoring that medical professionals need to do can now be performed on laptops. It's vastly improved over the last couple of years."

I would sit in his room every day and look at all the machinery. I got to know the staff, technician, and the Doctors, very well. One of the Technicians that cared for him most of the time was nicknamed Mad Dog. He was a fascinating man. We talked every day, and he explained what was going on with the equipment. I asked him many questions about the readings on the equipment. I am one of these people if I do not know something, I ask. Mad Dog was very patient with me.

Each day he had a different nurse as they work twelve-hour shifts so I would see them three days a week. Several were good about keeping me informed. There was one male nurse who was a pain in the rear, he would not tell me anything. He stayed with Cody even when he was out of the coma.

They had told me, people in a coma; know you are there, so you should talk to them. Therefore, I would talk to Cody every day, telling him what was going on in my life and at home. Telling him about the animals, etc. As it turned out, he did not even know I was there. I guessed medically induced comas are different than from a head trauma.

Some days it looked like things were going well with him and then bam it would go to shit. I probably drove the hospital nuts, with my questions, but I believe it saved Cody life in the end.

It is hard to go through a major change in your life in a State and City where you know no one. Cody's sister and brother-in-law were a great help, but they could not be there every day, as they worked. I had to grow whether I wanted to or not. However, one thing I learned, I hated the Denver traffic and driving Cody's car.

Throughout the whole situation, I ate, as I am a stress eater, I gained sixty pounds in the nine months we were in Denver. I could not be unhappy as this procedure was much needed for Cody to live, but I was. I am not a selfish person, but I knew I had a breaking point. I was homesick and very lonely. As I said earlier, this procedure affects everyone. It is a life changing process.

All the time Cody was in the hospital, I took care of the RV, our pets and I found a job that I could do from the Motorhome. I would process sales at night on the computer for a vitamin company, so the job was perfect. We were maintaining two homes, one in Denver, and one in Nevada. Therefore, the cost of all of this was affecting our budget. The Insurance Company paid for some things; like the RV rent, but not everything.

My Nevada family was watching our home and sending us our mail. However, there were bills to be paid for maintaining that house while living in the RV. It was interesting as I tried to figure out how to make it all work out here and at home. I miss my State and family. As I said, this illness affected everyone. Life changes a lot for everyone.

As I have stated about the e-mails, I wrote them every day for family and friends and for me to vent, while Cody was recovering. Please excuse the errors as I stated earlier, but they are the original emails. Many times, while typing, I could hardly see the keyboard because I was crying so much. The emails will give you a sense of what was happening during this process. I tried to sound upbeat, but still keeping everyone informed. I also called the hospital every evening to see how he was doing.

Date: Thu, 13 Jul 2006 14:47:59 -0700 (PDT)
Subject: Thur- Cody

Well, today was better, he is still in guarded status, but no more blood transfusions. His heart is still erratic, but nothing like yesterday. Today he is on 60% oxygen with Nitrous; they do not believe the breathing tube will be removed today. I did not get to see the Dr though I was there for several hours, but those Drs. are so busy.

So I am going to keep a positive thought that maybe the worst is over. He may be a few days behind, but who cares, we are not in a contest.

I think the news today was better than yesterday, he is not perfect, but it will happen.

What is Nitrous: The purpose of the machine allows for it to deliver a mixture of nitrous oxide and oxygen for the patient to inhale, in order to depress the feeling of pain while keeping the patient in a conscious state.

In Cody's case, he was in a coma but still felt some limited pain from the transplant.

I would then come home and take care of the animals. I was not sleeping very well. I would have nightmares about what if something happens to him. One day I came home with a bucket of KFC, I ate the whole bucket and did not even know I ate it. I started buying little bottles of booze and wine and having one each night, hoping they would help me sleep. Life was not good in "Mudville." However, when you are going through all of this, how do you complain and sound ungrateful.

I was happy for Cody but was unhappy at the same time. I believe this is known as depression, so if you every go through the transplant process, be prepared for these feelings, unless you have a support team close by.

Date: Fri, 14 Jul 2006 13:18:33 -0700 (PDT)

Subject: Friday Update on Cody

First, he looks good his coloring is good. The lungs are doing well, Dr. Z performed a test this morning, and they are coming along fine.

He is in a little above guarded condition. His

heart is still giving them fits. Cody is still on the ventilator; his oxygen now is at 55% and 45% him. He had a bad last night, got another pint of blood, and he is on medicine to slow the heart. The nurse said they may start to wean him today/evening on the drugs, to see how the heart does, but doubtful they will remove the ventilator.

This family has never done anything by the book, so what is going on does not alarm me. We just take one day at a time and pray that each day will get better. We knew the heart would be an issue, but Cody didn't have enough time to wait for the double lung and heart, so we will deal with this.

Keep him in your prayers, and this too shall pass.

I tried to sound strong in my e-mails, but I did not sleep well, and I ate too much. However, enough about me, this story is about the transplant. You learn to take one day at a time.

+++

Date: Sat, 15 Jul 2006 13:19:13 -0700 (PDT) "
Subject: Sat- Cody

This life-changing event has been an emotional roller coaster. Illness buts humble us, frustrates us and we learn to be patience and of course, I have no patience. I want him well now!

About 6:30 last night, they turned Cody off, and his oxygen levels plummeted. They upped the ventilator to 60%, took X-rays, gave some drugs, and got him stable by around 10. They placed him back on the lactic drip, as they want to drain more fluids. He has remained stable. Like I said yesterday, his color is good and is looking stronger.

Today, they cut back the NOX (nitrous), by 10 - whatever that means, so far no blood transfusions and they turned him with no problems. I do not know if I told everyone, but when they did the lung surgery, they did have to remove a lobe off one lung due to damage, and I guess when he is turned on that side, it gives them fits. He is off the lactic drip and just receiving shots, but he is still peeing like a racehorse. This is good.

They are hoping to remove some tubes today, and they are bringing him out of the medically-induced coma- this will take several days. He opened his eyes and understood who he was, but boy, his he stoned. Hee hee. They do not want to excite the body especially the heart. It is still erratic but is not spiking, which is good.

He will probably be in ICU for another few days

and then transferred to a private room. Normally he should have been out if ICU by now, walking and getting ready for rehab, so we are a little behind, but like I said before, this is one contest we can lose, and I am so glad the Dr's are taking their time.

I have not talked to Dr. Z for a couple of days, did talk today to a female Dr., don't remember her name. She was the one that said they might remove some of the tubes. He looks like a Sci-fi- Frankenstein right now, there are tubes everywhere.

So I think overall we are over the major humps, just a few more twist, and turns before the ride ends.

*ICU means Critical Care Unit.

Another day of watching him and wondering is he out of the woods. I would ask the nurses and technicians. They gave him enough drugs to keep him in the coma that they would fill up one of those needle containers a day.

Date: Sun, 16 Jul 2006 14:14:34 -0700 (PDT)

Subject: Sun - Cody

Well, that emotional roller coaster took a plunge again.

Early this morning, Cody took a dive and we are back at square one. His heart is the main problem, extremely erratic. He is in a full medically induced coma, on 70% oxygen from the ventilator (he was at

45%) and the NOX which was 5 is back to 20. He is running a fever and has an infection/pneumonia. So they have him on all kinds of medication. Too soon, to consider rejection, but they will watch the fever like mad.

The only good news at this point is he is bouncing back. At 7 am, he was on 100% ventilator and now he on 70%, so that is a good sign. The other good thing at this point, no more blood transfusions.

At 2 pm today, his vitals were stable. So we pray all is well in the next 24 hours. Will keep you informed.

"**Lung transplant (LT) recipients** are particularly susceptible to pneumonia in comparison with other solid organ transplant (SOT) recipients or similarly immunosuppressed patients. In addition to the generalized immunosuppression by antirejection medications, the lung allograft is denervated, the cough reflex is depressed, mucociliary clearance is decreased, and lymphatic drainage is disrupted. Pneumonia is a major cause of morbidity and mortality in LT recipients and mortality for pneumonia is higher in this group of patients than in other SOT recipients.

The etiology of pneumonia in LT patients is very varied and includes opportunistic, and hospital acquired microorganisms. The clinical symptoms and signs are frequently modified by the immunosuppression therapy.

Antimicrobial therapy is limited by the interactions with immunosuppressants and a higher incidence of adverse events, determining a poor prognosis. Prompt diagnosis and treatment are necessary to prevent poor outcomes.

An understanding of the temporal relationship between LT, the beginning of immunosuppression and the risk of developing pneumonia of different aetiologies may assist the appropriate treatment.

The probability of survival during the first year of follow-up was significantly higher in the multivariate analysis in LT recipients who did not have a pneumonia episode compared with those that had at least one episode" (CU

Cody has pneumonia, which is not a good thing, but we just had to ride it out.

Date: Mon, 17 Jul 2006 12:43:06 -0700 (PDT

Subject: Cody - Monday

Well, today, Cody's roller coaster ride is climbing back up and God I hope at the top is a curve and not another plunge.

The ventilator is now at 50%; they have removed some tubes from his stomach and are feeding him a liquid diet. As fussy as Cody is about his food, it is a good thing he is in a coma! The NOX has been lowered to 12. Believe these two items won't change anymore for a couple of days, they want to keep him stable, but they needed to have these new lungs working.

Other than that, he is still at square one. He does have an infection (pneumonia), but currently no fever he broke that yesterday. They did give another pint of blood. I talked to the Surgeon today and they are concerned about the infection, so he is in a critical state, but Cody is not in a critical condition. What that means, he is very sick, but stable.

Pray that this condition last for 36-48 hours, then they can start to bring him out of the coma. If anything changes will let you know.

Cody has now been a week in this condition. They had told us he would be in a coma for two to three days... Not. He is still in bad shape and in the medically induced coma.

Thank goodness for some friends in the Park. I cried every night. I come home from the hospital, walk the dogs, eat more than I should, I am gaining weight. I am so lonely, all of my family is back in Nevada, I talk and e-mail, but I could really use a big hug. Cody's family is thirty miles away, and I did not see them every day, usually once a week. Therefore, I would go down and cry on Susie's shoulder -- the owner of the park, and eat! I knew our life would never be the same. So Susie became my adopted Colorado daughter; I still love her to this day.

Date: Tue, 18 Jul 2006 12:28:55 -0700 (PDT)

Subject: Tues - Cody

Things are looking up; believe we may be getting off this rollercoaster ride.

Cody is off the NOX - first time ever. His ventilator is at 40%. The lungs are still wet, so they giving him stuff to dry out plus the lactic.

His coloring looks good. He is still in the medically induced coma, and they have not even tried to bring him out yet. He still has an infection in the lung, but no fever. The heart is stable between 58-65, and his oxygen level is great 93-98. It has been 48 hrs since the last dive, so believe we are going around the bend to recovery.

Thanks for all your prayers and kind thoughts.

One thing I learned throughout this whole process is to take one day at a time. I did not feel Cody was going to die, I just did not know when he would get better, if ever. Stress caused by a loved one's illness is hard to take, or at least it was for me. You can do whatever you want to me, but not my family. I do not like seeing my love ones suffer or be ill.

Date: Wed, 19 Jul 2006 12:36:23 -0700 (PDT)

Subject: Wed- Cody

Today, they are trying to bring him out of the medically-induced coma. He is agitated, and his heart is spiking, so they are monitoring him real careful. If he response well, they will remove him off the ventilator and start using a c-Pac machine.

The pneumonia is still there, they are clearing out the gunk. However, no fever and no additional blood transfusions. So overall, Cody is holding his own. Now we wait and take one day at a time. Each day, as you can tell, was an adventure, you never knew what to expect. I know all would be okay and all of this would be worth it. At least that is what I told myself that every day...

+++

Date: Thu, 20 Jul 2006 13:19:11 -0700 (PDT

Subject: Thur - Cody

The latest chapter.

Cody is doing OK, they had to up his ventilator from 40 to 80, but while I was there, they lowered to 70, maybe this evening back to 50%. I guess last night he took a dive on his oxygen levels. They took x-rays and everything seemed to be OK. When his fever spikes or his oxygen levels drop, they get concerned about rejection. But so far, everything seems OK.

He is agitated today, his pulse and heart erratic. But the good news, the pneumonia looks good and no blood transfusions. He is coming out of the medically induced coma, in fact, they have to tie his hands down, so, he won't pull out his tubes. He is not a happy camper right now, cannot blame him with a tube down your throat.

So that is about it for now.

Keep your fingers crossed that we have passed all the bad stuff and everything is getting better, that was what I was telling myself every day.

Date: Sat, 22 Jul 2006 14:20:22 -0700 (PDT)

Subject: Sat- Cody's update.

Day Eleven: Well, things are about the same, his fever is back, but low. They gave him another pint of blood, that is 9, but the good news is the ventilator is at 40%. He can move but is still sedated, so not coming out of the coma.

While I was typing this, the Dr. called, and his stats dropped, and they are upping the ventilator. The Dr. said if we can get rid of the pneumonia, everything else will fall into place. He would like him out of the coma within the next week, so we will see. According to Dr. L, his stats drop because of the pneumonia, as his new lungs are looking good. They will not take him fully off the ventilator until he is out of the coma, so he knows to breathe and cough. Every time, they try to bring him out, the heart goes crazy.

The pneumonia looks good one day and back the next. Today, it is better, so who knows. I just worry that he has the strength to keep up with all of this.

They cannot keep him in a coma for too long, or other damages occur. So we watch and wait.

Date: Sun, 23 Jul 2006 12:46:38 -0700 (PDT

Twelfth day in ICU: Fever is gone; pneumonia is a little better, now he has extra fluid on the outside of the lung. This is nothing out of the normal, as they have two tubes draining now, but may have to add a third.

Every day is a challenge, he is still sedated but can move and does it a lot, and he is coughing, which is good. The Dr wants to get him up as soon as possible, as every day he is sedated, he gets weaker. But can't get him off the sedation till he gets better. The circle.

After twelve days, Cody has not improved overall, but God willing he will. I won't send any more updates, until I have some consistent news, because at this point the news goes from bad to good; back to bad. And this just upsets us all. Today he is holding his own considering the above.

Something is wrong, I can feel it, but not sure what. I asked the technician Mike, he said things should have leveled out by now. When Bob and Mary came to visit, I asked what they thought. They thought he looked fine.

Date: Mon, 24 Jul 2006 14:40:16 -0700 (PDT)

Subject: Mon-Cody

Thirteenth day: I said I wasn't going to send any more updates, unless some good news. Today news was a change.

From 8 - 10 this morning, he was breathing on his own. He is back on the ventilator at 40%, not sure why they put him back on. They are bringing him out of the sedated coma, hope it works this time. They did a bronshopy (spelled wrong) at 10, then sent Cody for X-rays and a cat scan, I have not heard the results of those tests, but do know they place him back on lactic and another drug to make him pee.

It will take several days for him to come completely out of the coma. There will be memory loss, how much, not sure. He still has lots of infection, and that may be the reason for the c-scan as well as the meds to get rid of the fluids, who knows. Even the nurse didn't know.

By the time I left, he was becoming agitated and moving a lot. His heart rate was good, but he is medicated. So let's hope he has reached the turning point.

I gave the info to the Nurse to give to the Dr., as I never saw him, but the nurse said he was swamped. The Dr. is supposed to call later this afternoon. Things are not right.

That is it for now.

Now two weeks have gone by, and I don't see positive changes. I talked to Dr. L that afternoon, I said I felt things are not going well. I watch Cody every day, something is wrong, he is not getting any better. In fact, he is getting worse. He said they were going to run some more test. I complained that he had been in a coma for two weeks. He explained it was because of the heart. I did not buy it.

The next evening he called and said, "We're going to have to do another surgery. Would I give my consent, it was a high-risk surgery as, after the lung examination, they found a hole in his new lungs."

I laughed nervously and said, "Yes, he is not going to make it the way he is?"

The Doctor further reiterated how serious this surgery would be.

Again, I laughed nervously, "and what we have been going through is not serious?"

Needless to say, I didn't make brownie points with the Dr. L. However, it rather ticked me off that I had to bring it to his attention that something was wrong. We had come too far to fail now.

I know the Dr. was trying to forewarn me that Cody could die during this surgery. I was well aware of the choice I had just made. I was so upset when I got off the phone with the Doctor, *what if I made the wrong decision??* I am a strong person and used to making hard decisions, but this was different. I was so stressed; I ate some chocolate mint cookies and drank a little bottle of margarita, what a combination. I got dreadful heartburn, but didn't care, and I cried and cried.

One of the people in the park came by to see how I was doing; as I was a slobbering mess. He listened to me and said I did the right thing. However, it still did not help my heartburn, or how I felt about the decision.

It was a long night.

Chapter Eight - Second Surgery and Final Recovery.

Here are the e-mails regarding the second surgery and his recovery.

Date: Tue, 25 Jul 2006 16:07:53 -0700 (PDT)

Tuesday -Number 14.

We are waiting to go into surgery. Dr. L said it could be this evening or tomorrow... It is now 5:00 pm here so; I assume the surgery will be tomorrow. Cody has a hole and infection in the new lung. When it was installed there was some damage to one lobe, which was operated on. Due to the pneumonia and coughing, he has disturbed the surgery on his lung, and it is infected. This is a major setback.

Today, they had Cody off the ventilator and breathing on a c-pack. He still has the tube in this throat. He is coming out of the coma and could answer some questions. Everything is good except now we have to go back in. This new surgery will be 2-4 hours.

Will keep you informed.

I am hoping all goes well and this is the light before the dawn... I am not sure I can take much more stress.

Date: Wed, 26 Jul 2006 09:25:14 -0700 (PDT)

Subject: Wed-Cody

Just a quick note to say we go for the lung repair surgery on the infected lung tentative at 6: p.m. Colorado time. It will take from two to four hours. Cody had a good day yesterday, so let's hope that good luck continues. I am going into the hospital around 4 p.m. as right now he is sedated. They want him to rest for the surgery.

Bob is taking me to the hospital, as I am such a wimp about driving freeways at night or in lots of traffic, so God bless Bob. Will email with the news of the surgery.

That is it for now

Bob sat with me in the same waiting room as before. The same waiting room with the coffee table filled with tattered magazines and travel books, cardboard holders with pamphlets, advertisement posters on the walls, and hallway leading to operating rooms. TV's were playing in all four corners of the large room.

Again, we waited while Cody went through this surgery. Mary was out of town for work. This surgery only took three to four hours. The doctor that performed Cody's surgery was the most handsome man I have ever seen. I could hardly concentrate on what he was saying, as he was so handsome.

I told Cody that was the best thing that had happened through this whole adventure. We still laugh and talked about it today; that man could have eaten crackers in my bed...

Date: Wed, 26 Jul 2006 23:14:37 -0700 (PDT)

Subject: Cody - surgery

Well, the surgery went well; the Dr accomplished everything that had to be done.

His heart and pulse did fine, everything went well. We need to get him up as soon as possible, cause if stays on the ventilator too much longer, they may have to go in and do a third surgery. He still has pneumonia; they did take some gunk out and added two more drain tubes to help get the fluids off the lungs.

Now we wait and see. I will see him in the morning and will send an update after the visit.

Thanks for your prayers,

Keep your finger crossed that this surgery works. We need some good luck right now.

Date: Thu, 27 Jul 2006 13:44:38 -0700 (PDT)

Subject: Thur- Cody

Day 16:

Best day as of yet.

Cody is alert, they removed the tube, and he can whisper. Stats are looking good. He still has pneumonia, but it is looking better. He is weak, but hell, who wouldn't be after two major surgeries. Last night surgery was 3 1/2 hrs. So hopefully this roller coaster ride we have been on is coming into the station, and we can get off!

So that is it, for now, thank you so much for all your prayers, but don't stop, we still aren't out of the woods, but we can see the clearing. Wahoo. The tides are turning, I did my happy dance.

Date: Fri, 28 Jul 2006 13:16:31 -0700 (PDT)

Subject: Cody- Fri

Fri Update:

Things are going great. He is talking, said he had the shit beat out of him, and he is right. He is breathing on his own. So life is good!

Date: Sat, 29 Jul 2006 13:54:21 -0700 (PDT)

Subject: Sat- Cody

Each day is better, can't believe how he has changed. He is still coming out of the medicated coma; will take a few more days. He is starting to complain, so you know he is feeling better. He started eating today - liquid diet at this time, but he is eating.

He still has some pneumonia, but it is just about gone. So that is it for now.

"It was like, just yesterday I was dying, I could barely breathe, and today, I'm breathing like a normal person again," he said. *"It took a few days to set in. Every day I would wake up and slowly breath and think, 'Is this for real?"* This quote from another double lung transplant recipient.

+++

Date: Sun, 30 Jul 2006 16:00:48 -0700 (PDT)
Subject: Sun Cody

Cody is doing great at this point. I cannot believe the difference from last Sunday until now.

Dr. L told Cody today that the Wed. Surgery was a major setback, and it will be a long road to recovery. He still has an infection, but it is under control. Today they had him in a chair, he is too weak to get up, they roll him onto this chair then elevate. He ate real people food and did quite well. He is too weak to feed himself; in fact, he can't raise his hands to scratch his nose. But he is getting stronger each day. He cried when I came in, and I tease him that he must have got a set of sensitive lungs. He read some cards that were sent, and he cried, so I am suspicious... smile.

Right before I left, he was tired, so they put him back to bed, said they would get him up again tonight. So we take one day at a time, as there is sunshine at the end of this road.

The next day when I came to visit him, he asked why I had never been to see him in the hospital. I said "What, I have been here every day since the surgery. I am the one that found out you needed a second surgery." I was angry, then hurt and pissed.

I was hurt that he was angry with me. We talked about this incident, even now; I have never forgiven him for those remarks. I tried to justify the remarks, that it was the medication he was taking. However, even, after all these years, it still has not helped. The thing that still hurts is it was all about him. He never asked how I did, why he was in the hospital. Guess that is the selfish part of me to think that way, but my life was in turmoil too.

Date: Mon, 31 Jul 2006 14:08:08 -0700 (PDT)

Subject: Mon - Cody

Day 20.

Well, today was not a good day. They placed him in his chair, and he is eating, I fed him, as he cannot feed himself. He didn't like the Dr., isn't pleased with the lungs, you name it, etc. He is grumpy, so much, for the sensitive sides... smile.

The concerns today are as follows:

Pulmonary edema, they did a bronchscopy (spelled wrong) this morning, and his lungs are wet again, so he is back on pee medicine. This is not pneumonia. They are not sure if the stuff they took out this morning is infected, but will know by this afternoon. He is taking an antibacterial medicine, and they added potassium. So he is still on IV's. He still has three drain tubes from the chest, and they are draining.

He is extremely disoriented and tells stories. They did not give us a report yet on what was wrong with his old lungs. Today he was mad at me for not driving him home, couldn't remember where he was and wanted to eat outside, stuff like that. The Nurse says it is not normal behavior, but also not out of the ordinary either for the length of time he was in the coma.

His oxygen levels were up from 1 liter to 4, and when they moved him, he plummeted to 70, mainly because of the fluid in his lungs. The long and short of this, each day we take one day at a time, pray, and hope the lungs are taking. Both Dr.'s said it would be a long road to recovery.

Hell, tomorrow I will write, he is up and dancing down the hall - who knows what 24 hours will bring.

"What is Pulmonary edema; is a buildup of fluid in the lung that limits breathing. Pulmonary edema can be serious and life-threatening.

The most common cause of pulmonary edema is heart

disease or heart failure, which prevents the heart from pumping effectively and leads to fluid buildup in the lungs and other parts of the body. Damage to the lungs themselves can also cause pulmonary edema. Such damage may be the result of trauma, inhaled toxins, infection, or some medications."

Date: Tue, 1 Aug 2006 15:14:17 -0700 (PDT)

Subject: Tues - Cody

Well, it has been 3 weeks since the transplant surgery, and things are going well.

Cody wasn't dancing in the halls today, he is still disoriented. He was mad at me because I don't come to visit him and I won't take him home. In fact, the nurse said tonight when I call she will put him on the phone. She said this behavior will pass with time.

Heath wise about the same, still getting rid of fluids. He ate well today, best so far. He has a change in Dr's, Dr. Joe is now his Dr. We started this process with him, and he is a good Doctor. Dr. L was transferred to another facility. Cody is still weak, can't feed himself yet.

So that is it, for now, again thank you for your support and prayers.

I did not understand nor do I till this day, why he was so mad at me. He said it was because when he came out of the coma, he did not know where he was, what was going on.

I try to keep that in mine, but it is hard.

Date: Sun, 6 Aug 2006 20:59:58 -0700 (PDT)

Subject: Sun - Cody

Cody was moved last night from ICU to a private room. He is still real weak and can't walk, but he is doing better. He still has a drainage tube, and numerous IV's but is in a good mood, says he will be up and out in ten days, so let's pray. He has a phone in his room. So we are now in the meadow, still having some woods to get through, but things are looking good.

So each day things get better.

We are on the road to recovery, thank goodness. I want to go home to Nevada...

Date: Thu, 10 Aug 2006 13:23:50 -0700 (PDT)

Subject: Thur - Cody

News of today: Cody is waiting on the insurance to be transferred to rehab for 3-4 days to build his strength. He has a rattle back in his lungs, so he is back on anti-bacterial medicine. He can sit up real good, eat well and was able to get up today with the walker and make a couple of steps. They may take him off the oxygen today. Still, has neck tubes. Compare to last week this time he has improved 100%. He has now been in the hospital 32 days. Not bad for two major surgeries. Figure he might get out next Fri, all depends, but we want him well when he gets out.

Let's hope he gets to get out, he is still grumpy. The time spent in the hospital is not as pleasant as when he was in the coma. Now I get to listen to him bitch. His glass is still half-empty.

Date: Thu, 17 Aug 2006 19:01:50 -0700 (PDT)

Subject: Cody - Thur

This is the latest:

This evening they moved Cody to rehab. So he has a new phone number. He will be there at least until Monday, if all goes well, he will be sent home, if not, they will keep him longer.

They removed his staples, had about 100. Yesterday his heart was acting up and was back on IV's, but removed those this evening. He only uses oxygen when he walks and then only 1-2 liters, so he is doing great there, we just need to get his strength up.

That's it for now.

While in Rehab Cody suspected he may have

had a little stroke while in the coma, we will never know for sure, but rehab was hard on him. Nevertheless, with new lungs, you have to exercise.

Date: Tue, 22 Aug 2006 13:43:41 -0700 (PDT)

Subject: Cody

Well, it is planned that Cody will be released tomorrow from the hospital. He has been in over 6 weeks. I won't have to drive to Denver every day anymore. I hate Denver traffic. Bob is helping me to bring him home. He will be on a walker and oxygen only when needed. So life is good.

What can I say wahoo I will not have to drive to Denver every day...?

Date: Wed, 23 Aug 2006 16:27:34 -0700 (PDT)

Subject: Cody

Cody is home.

Over the next few days, he was doing well, walking the park with the dogs, going to the store. He refuses to wear his mask, again does not want people to notice him. Not using any oxygen, as the lungs are working. He has tons of medicine to take each day. He has said a couple of time if he knew what this surgery entailed, he really has to think about doing it again. We both knew as we had the training to understand the procedures. He wanted to live, and he would do it again.

Date: Fri, 8 Sep 2006 16:46:14 -0700 (PDT)
Subject: Cody

Well, we should not have bragged about how good Cody was doing. Cody is going back into the hospital tonight for at least five days. He caught some kind of virus, not sure how. Will keep you informed about what is happening.

"What is Human rhinovirus; is a leading cause of respiratory infections in adults and children. Adults, on average, get infected with the virus once per year. Lung transplant patients, with impaired immune systems due to drugs to halt rejection, are at potentially higher risk from the virus.

"Our evidence demonstrates that rhinoviral disease is not exclusively limited to the upper respiratory tract," said Dr. Kaiser. "It can also lead to lower respiratory complications, which immunosuppressed patients can be at higher risk of developing."

Although eight lung transplant patients had transient rhinoviral infections, three showed a persistent infection. The others were able to clear the virus from their system.

"We confirmed the persistence of a single strain in each of three lung transplant recipients clinically infected by rhinovirus," said Dr. Kaiser. "Two of the three had chronic upper respiratory tract infections. All three had relapsing lower respiratory infections, and two subsequently died with graft dysfunction."

Dr. Kaiser noted that the persistent infection suggests that certain cases can act as viral reservoirs to sustain transmission of rhinovirus.

"Therefore, in lung transplant recipients with severe immunosuppression, clinical rhinovirus infection needs to be considered," said Dr. Kaiser. "This point might have substantial implications in terms of diagnostic procedures, clinical management, and antiviral use, if available."

Date: Sun, 10 Sep 2006 17:48:05 -0700 (PDT)
Subject: Cody

As I told you on Friday, Cody is back in the hospital, he has a virus and is on Ribavirin treatments, they administer it by aerosol mist through a ventilator three times a day, for five days and it takes two hours to be administered. He is feeling fine, just tired. They said he will feel worse before it is over and we are praying these treatments will take care of this and he won't be in the hospital longer. Other than that, he has improved greatly. He can walk really well now and is not on any air. They told us we would have these bumps in the road, they just didn't expect it this quick.

Hey, life is like a soap opera, and we just have to learn to take one day at a time.

This was nothing out of the ordinary to get this virus in new lung transplant patients. But both of us were tired. We wanted to get our lives back to some normalcy. Cody has since gotten the rhinovirus several more times. He has nine lives.

Date: Wed, 20 Sep 2006 16:02:45 -0600

Subject: Cody on Sunday

Well, Cody got out of the hospital today and is doing Ok. So we will take one day at a time. Thanks for all your kind thoughts.

Chapter Nine – Waiting to go Back to Nevada

"Lung Transplant Prognosis: A lung transplant can take away breathlessness and make possible an active lifestyle that can last for years. For many people, a lung transplant is nothing less than lifesaving.

After recovering from lung transplant surgery, more than 80% of the people say they have no limitations on their physical activity. Among people surviving five years or more, up to 40% continue to work at least part time." (CU)

During research on many sites, I found this information. Eventual complications after lung transplant are inevitable. The immune system's rejection of the new lungs can be slowed, but not stopped entirely. In addition, the necessary powerful immune-suppressing drugs have unavoidable side effects, including diabetes, kidney damage, and vulnerability to infections, we knew we would have to live with this.

For these reasons, long-term survival after a lung transplant is not as promising as it is after other organ transplants, like kidney or liver.

Still, more than 80% of people survive at least one year after lung transplant. After three years, between 55% and 70% of those receiving lung transplants are alive. Age at the time of transplant is the most important factor influencing lung transplant survival. Cody has made eleven years.

+++

Over time, Cody felt so good not having to have oxygen from a tank or concentrator. We wandered around Colorado, getting to see the State. The hospital would not release him to go back to Nevada just yet.

+++

It was the start of a beautiful fall. Colorado has an awesome Fall with all the colors of the trees. We went to South Park, rode the train at George Town and visited several ghost towns one being Leadville. Majestic mountains and breathtaking scenic views surround the other ghost town of Cripple Creek, which is located at the base of Pikes Peak, the historic mining town. The boom of Colorado's Gold Rush puts Cripple Creek on the map. More than 100 years ago, this mining community attracted thousands of gold-seekers in search of their fortunes, and you can still do, that there today in the towns casinos and gaming halls, the same as Black Hawk and Central City.

We traveled to Boulder, which is a college town, it is tucked into a picturesque valley below the iconic Flatirons. Boulder hosts thriving tech, and natural food industries support a renowned entrepreneurial community, has some of the region's best restaurants, and is home to many federal research labs and an excellent university. This Rocky Mountain town is a wonderful destination. They have great shops and beer pubs. Boulder has become a "foodie town." You can grab a bite to eat at any one of the many award-winning restaurants. In Boulder alone, there are dozens of some of the country's finest microbrews. We had to try a few. Yes, Cody could drink in moderation.

Then we took a day and drove to the Garden of the Gods in Colorado Springs. This is a beautiful place of carved rocks, was a nice hike and Tom did not have to pack oxygen. There are fifteen miles of trails that wind through the park and range from easy loops to moderate 3-milers. The paved Perkins Central Garden Trail is a favorite of those just out for a stroll and is wheelchair- and stroller-accessible. Playing tourist was healing for both of us.

We visited Golden, which was a short distance from Wheatridge. Golden has a small town charm that comes with great recreation, including hiking, mountain biking, and water sports. There is cultural attractions, affordable dining, and eclectic shopping. The main attraction is the world's largest single-site brewery, the Coors Brewery Tour. We tried a few of their new beers for fun.

Golden is a place of history mixed with contemporary fun. You can experience the Old West at the historic Clear Creek History Park, climb aboard the trains at the Colorado

Railroad Museum. At the time, I was active in the Virginia and Truckee Railroad, so the Museum was a must to see. Both Cody and I love railroads.

We rode the Georgetown Railroad Loop. Georgetown was a silver mining camp along Clear Creek in the Front Range of the Rocky Mountains. It was established in 1859 during the Pike's Peak Gold Rush. Today, the federally designated Georgetown-Silver Plume National Historic District comprises Georgetown, the nearby Town of Silver Plume, and the Georgetown Loop Historic Mining & Railroad Park between the two towns. The town is nestled in the mountains near the upper end of the valley of Clear Creek. It is a small town today, when we were there, they had snow.

We travel the Lariat Loop, which featuring Buffalo Bill's Grave and Museum on Lookout Mountain. Cody's Great-Great Uncle was Buffalo Bill. Therefore, we had to go to his gravesite. "Where the West Lives!

We also traveled to Estes Park. The town is a popular summer resort and the location of the headquarters for Rocky Mountain National Park, Estes Park lies along the Big Thompson River. Landmarks include the Stanley Hotel. The Stanley Hotel, known for its architecture, magnificent setting, and famous visitors, best known today for its inspirational role in the Stephen King's novel, "The Shining." This hotel has been featured as one of America's most haunted hotel, with the numerous stories from visitors and staff, The Stanley Hotel continues to "shine" today, as it did in 1909 when first opened. We were able to climb around the Hotel property, it was awesome.

Nevada is a gambling State; it is not in Colorado except in a couple counties. They have taken old mining towns and made them into gambling places.

"Cripple Creek played an integral role in the rich heritage of Colorado. In 1890, a ranch hand named Bob Womack discovered gold and Cripple Creek changed forever. By 1900, more than 50,000 people called the gold camp home. When the golden era ended in 1918, more than $300 million in gold had been mined in what would be the last great gold rush in North America.

By the 1920s, only about 40 mines remained. However, two decades later, in the 1940s, the town began to promote itself as a tourist destination, offering visitors a glimpse into the past. (Wikepedia)

In 1991, the town was opened to limited-stakes gaming. Today, the old gold camp has reinvented itself as a full-service tourist destination with many gambling houses, all the while preserving and showcasing its rich history. They look like mining camps on the outside, but inside they are gaming houses.

We also went to Leadville. A former silver mining town

that lies near the headwaters of the Arkansas River. Located in the heart of the Rocky Mountains. Elevation 10,152. Colorado has some high mountain towns.

All the places we went to were interesting, good food, and great shops, we had fun. Colorado is a beautiful State, too many people for my taste, as everywhere you went you saw a rooftop.

Date: Sat, 21 Oct 2006 09:54:32 -0700

Subject: Update on Cody

We ran into a few snags. The good news is they have released Cody, the bad news they have scheduled him for tests on 10/30 and 11 /13, plus they want to see him every 6 weeks for six months. On top of this we just had our second snow storm, so the plan is to leave on the 11/14 weather permitting and head home, then he can fly back (hopefully we will find cheap tickets) till spring, then we will drive back out. Also, we hope after six months, that he will only have to come back to Denver twice a year and we can live with that.

It was a good thing we didn't leave after his last bronk on Monday, as they found an infection Friday, which they jumped on ASAP. So he takes that medicine for seven days. The worst-case scenario is they may do another bronk to check on the right lung, which is the one that is giving him so many problems. The right lung was the one with a little damage. It caused the second surgery and pneumonia.

Other than that he is walking 2-3 miles a day, weather permitting, poor Dakota (the dog) is getting skinny and Cody has a lot of energy. We are hoping to be home by Thanksgiving, so keep your fingers crossed.

I am working 40+ hours a week, wasn't part of the plan, was to be 25 hours, but my boss has been ill. Love the job though, all computer work and some phones here in the motor home. The commute to work though is killer... smile.

Well, that is it, for now, Have a great Halloween, we miss you all.

Chapter Ten - Going Home

Date: Mon, 13 Nov 2006 17:09:48 -0800 (PST)
Subject: Going Home

Whoopee! We are going home!! Cody doesn't have to be back until Jan 8th; The Doctor extended the time due to the holidays. They do however want to see him every 6 weeks for the next 6 months. They are treating him as a high-risk patient. As the Dr. said today, we have too much time invested in him, and we want to make sure he succeeds. I personally agree!

We will break down the Motorhome tomorrow, though it is expected to snow, in fact, they have already received 10-18 inches in the mountain and it coming toward us for tonight, we are to receive 4 inches with high winds 40-50 mph. So we will try to leave Wed mid-morning, taking the southern route through New Mexico, Arizona and then come up through Vegas.

We plan to be home before Thanksgiving, weather willing. It is not fun to drive a hi-profile vehicle in the wind, so we will take it slow.

So maybe Tuesday tacos are coming for us next week. We miss everybody soooo much and just can't wait to get home!

Just wait to you see Cody, no trail of tanks. He is walking 5-6 miles a day, He looks great, and I look old, tired, and fat! My hair is really getting gray, but I am walking a mile or so a day.

See some of you soon. We will miss our Denver family, but we will be seeing them more than we ever did before.

Date: Wed, 15 Nov 2006 16:18:58 -0800 (PST

Subject: On our Way

Well, we are Raton, New Mexico on our way home. We only made 250 miles today, as we got a late start. Yesterday was so windy and cold couldn't finish breaking down the coach.

So today, we got the oil changes, etc. and left Wheatridge around 11:30 a.m... I didn't want to push too far as Cody is driving. It may take a little longer to come home, but that is OK. The weather today was good. The wind was nothing like yesterday.

We have wifi, so can receive mail tonight. Everyone is fine. We had an emotional day, going to miss the friends we made and family in CO and look forward to seeing friends and family in NV.

Date: Fri, 17 Nov 2006 15:25:14 -0800 (PST)

Subject: Trip Home

We are in Williams, Arizona, should make Pahrump-outside Vegas tomorrow and home Sunday.

Cody is doing great. Everything is going Ok, no troubles with R/V or car, so that is good. It is warm here in Williams, have the fans going. I like this area of AZ always have, we are right outside of the Grand Canyon and Route 66. We have stayed in this R/V Park before.

So that is it for now.

Date: Mon, 20 Nov 2006 18:04:40 -0800 (PST)

Subject: We are home

After over 8 months, we are home. The family and adopted family met us Sunday night when we got in around 8 pm, the first thing I did, after hugging and kissing the family, was to hug my counters, sink, washing machine and ice machine, ah the little things in life. Was a long day - was a long trip 1500 miles.

The grandbabies had grown a foot. The house looked so big after living in 250 sq. feet for the eight months. I woke up in the middle of the night and didn't know where I was. It is amazing how we adapt to our surroundings.

Cody is doing great and did well on the trip.

I cannot believe the amount of stuff we gather to bring home, we have boxes of non-important mail to go through, and it may take till Christmas to get caught up. I still have to get the paper and garbage service back up and running, all those little things you don't think about... The kids did a great job taking care of the house, now I just have all the little things I wanted to do before we left to do. Maybe I will get my kitchen finally finished (ha ha).

With Cody feeling so good, we are going to make some short trips, back in that motor home (smile). However, the first good day, we are off in the hot rod to visit friends. Sure did miss the hot rod, for those of you who don't know we have 1968 Chevelle SS396 besides the 1968 Charge R/T.

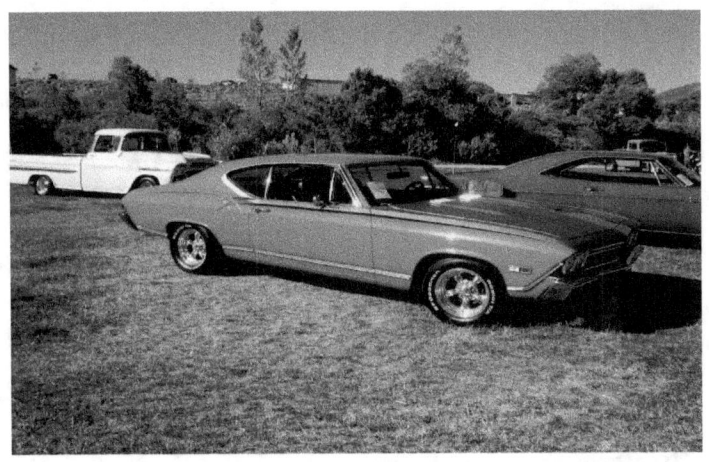

Cody went back to Denver January 8th for three days; he had to go back every 6 weeks for 6 months, then hopefully twice a year. I still cannot believe this was a man on death door and now he is walking 5-6 miles a day with his new lungs. Life is reborn!

Thanks so much to all of you for your understanding,

help, and support through this last eight months, I couldn't have done it without you. You are all the true meaning of friends and family!

Chapter Eleven – A Few Years that Followed

Well, how do you continue a story that you hopes has no ending. Cody is now eleven years out... not bad when they gave us three to five years.

+++

The first year after the surgery at home Cody was almost normal. He was unhappy that he had to take some many pills and go back to Denver every three months for a check-up. Overall, he did well and was feeling like his old self. He had a few minor hip-cups, but nothing serious. He caught a cold because he would not wear his mask in public. With no treating physicians in Nevada, every time he got sick, it was off to Denver.

Life was somewhat normal for us. We went on a cruise to Hawaii in February of 2007, and we were remarried on Valentine's Day. We called it his "Celebration of Life" cruise. He had a very good time, warm weather and we did not have to pack any oxygen. Cody may not show that he is happy with his new lungs, but he is. He always has to be so stotic. The cruise sailed round-trip from San Francisco for fifteen days and stopped at ports of call on Hawaii's Big Island, Oahu, Kauai, and Maui. The last stop on each of these cruises is in Ensenada, Mexico, before returning to the Port of San

Francisco. It was what we both needed.

We took in Pearl Harbor, home of the Japanese attack on Pearl Harbor and the United States' entry into World War II. It was quite a moving site to see. Pearl Harbor and the USS Arizona Memorial remain the most popular visitor attractions in Hawaii, with over 1,600,000 visitors annually.

On the morning of December 7, 1941, hundreds of Japanese fighter planes attacked the American naval base at Pearl Harbor near Honolulu. The surprise attack destroyed nearly 20 vessels, killed more than 2,000 American soldiers, and propelled the United States into World War II. Hawaii became the 50th U.S. state on August 21, 1959.

If fact, many of the passengers on the ship were world war two vets going back to see the museum. We meet several as they were at our dining table. The stories they could tell. However, by 9:00 p.m. the ship was dead, everyone had gone to bed. We met some crazy Canadians and partied into the night.

We took a bus tour of the Volcano. The Volcano is located on the border of Hawaii Volcanoes National Park and near the northeast rim of Kilauea's summit caldera. It was 80 degree at the base of the volcano and 40 degrees when we got to the top, in fact, it started to snow. We also saw the flow at night from the ship. It is an impressive sight.

We took a bus tour to Maui. The island of Maui is the

second-largest of the Hawaiian Islands at 727.2 square miles and is the 17th largest island in the United States. Maui is part of the State of Hawaii and is the largest of Maui County's four islands. Maui's diverse landscapes are the result of a unique combination of geology, topography, and climate. They had a great macadamia nut factory. I love the garlic flavored ones.

My favorite place was Kona for coffee, and it is dry like Nevada. In the Hawaiian language, Kona means leeward or dry side of the island, as opposed to ko'olau which means windward or the wet side of the island. In the times of Ancient Hawaii, Kona was the name of the Leeward district on each major island. In Hawai'i, the Pacific anticyclone provides moist prevailing northeasterly winds to the Hawaiian islands, resulting in rain when the winds contact the windward landmass of the islands - the winds subsequently lose their moisture and travel on to the leeward (or Kona) side of the island. When this pattern reverses, it can produce a Kona storm from the west.

We went to the big Island Hawaii; it was too big for me. Hawaii (Hawaiian: Hawai'i) is a group of volcanic islands in the central Pacific Ocean. The Islands lie 2,397 miles from San Francisco, California, to the east and 5,293 miles from Manila, in the Philippines, to the west. The capital is Honolulu, located on the island of Oahu. The islands were annexed by the United States in 1900, and as a U.S., territory saw population expansion and the establishment of a plantation system for growing sugar cane and pineapples.

While on the cruise we saw Waimea Canyon, also known as the Grand Canyon of the Pacific, is a large canyon, approximately ten miles long and up to 3,000 feet deep, located on the western side of Kauai in the Hawaiian Islands of the United States. Waimea is Hawaiian for "reddish water," a reference to the erosion of the canyon's red soil. The canyon was formed by a deep incision of the Waimea River arising from the extreme rainfall on the island's central peak, Mount Wai'ale'ale, among the wettest places on earth.

Geologically the canyon is carved into the tholeiitic and post-shield calc-alkaline lavas of the canyon basalt. The lavas of the canyon provide evidence for massive faulting and collapse in the early history of the island. The west side of the canyon is all thin, west-dipping lavas of the Nepali Member, while the eastern side is very thick, flat-lying lavas of the Olokele and Makaweli Members. The two sides are separated by an enormous fault along which a large part of the island moved downwards in a big collapse. It is not as big as stateside Grand Canyon, but it was magnificent.

We saw so many more sights. It was a great trip, and best of all, Cody did not have to pack oxygen.

+++

In 2008, Cody had to have surgery for Gastroesophageal

reflux disease (GERD). He had also gained about fifty pounds, from the medicine, even though he walked three to four miles a day and rode a bike.

"Gastroesophageal reflux disease (GERD) is thought to be a risk factor for the development or progression of chronic rejection after lung transplantation. However, the prevalence of GERD and its risk factors, including esophageal dysmotility, hiatal hernia, and delayed gastric emptying after lung transplantation, are still unknown."

They say it occurs, because of all the medicine he is taking. They had told us he would have problems from the meds and this was one of them. They also stated he would have trouble with his eyes, teeth, and bones. We went back to Denver for ten days for the surgery. I stayed with his family while he was in the hospital. The surgery went well. He still made his trips to Denver twice more that year for checkups.

2009 he was back in the hospital for a hernia surgery. This is the area below the abdomen, where part of the intestine has pushed through a tear in the muscle wall caused by a strain, such as lifting a heavy object. We are not sure why Cody got a hernia; it may have had something to do with the GERT. This surgery did not go so well. He developed an infection; remember he has no immune system. Cody had to wear a wound vacuum for thirty days.

"A wound VAC (vacuum assisted closure) is a device

which allows people to conduct negative pressure wound therapy (NPWT). The device consists of dressing, which is fitted with a tube and attached to the wound VAC. Negative pressure wound therapy is most commonly used with chronic wounds, which are not responding to other forms of treatment, and sometimes with surgical wounds, which have reopened. It usually requires the supervision of a nurse, although people do not need to be hospitalized to use a wound VAC". (CU)

Denver let us come home, and the local hospital maintained the cleaning of the wound VAC. Twice a week he would go to the local hospital for this procedure. This procedure cost us out of pocket-$30 a day and the cost of the wound VAC. He was on the wound VAC for about six weeks. Cody was not a happy camper as it is cumbersome to get around with and sleep. Finally, the wound healed and he was off the machine.

During 2010, we made five trips to Denver for hospital stays and infusion treatments. The medical cost just keeps piling up...

What is infusion therapy?

Infusion therapy involves the administration of medication through a needle or catheter. It is prescribed when a patient's condition is so severe that it cannot be treated effectively with oral medications. Typically, "infusion therapy" means that a drug is administered intravenously.

"Traditional" prescription drug therapies commonly administered via infusion include antibiotic, antifungal, antiviral, chemotherapy, hydration, pain management, and parenteral nutrition. (In Cody's case, it was steroids).

Infusion therapy is also provided to patients for treating a wide assortment of often chronic and sometimes rare diseases for which "specialty" infusion medications are effective.

Cody would have one treatment a day, for five days. He was high on steroids. All medications have risks of side effects, with some side effects being severe. If a person has been prescribed with steroids, he could be subject to wild mood swings, sometimes known as "roid rage." Then it would take a week or better to get the steroids out of his system. He basically was a drunk and irritable for a week. It also turned him a light pink. These treatments were done five times between 2010 and 2011 and remember each treatment is for five days. He also had the treatment in 2013, and three in 2014, in 2015 and 2016. He even started off 2017 of this year with treatment. It is used to stop lung rejection.

In between all of this, we did several more cruises to Panama and a couple to Alaska. The Panama cruise was on both of our bucket lists. The canal is an engineering feat in itself. We first flew to Florida and met our daughter, son in law and granddaughter. We spend five days at Disney world and Universal Studios. They went home, and we caught the cruise.

A dream more than 400 years in the making, the Panama Canal opened in 1914, and this epic man-made marvel changed the world in the process. There is no better way to discover this colossal wonder than on a Panama Canal cruise. Sail between two mighty oceans or sail a partial transit round-trip from Ft. Lauderdale, and discover why Condé Nast Traveler named it among its top "Where To Go" attractions. Expert narration enlightens as our ship passed through the locks, and you dined on authentic Panamanian cuisine. Ashore there is everything from Costa Rican rainforests to Old World cities like Cartagena that recall the Age of Exploration. The best part we saw it all, we went to Costa Rico and drank beer on the beach in Nicaragua, shopped in Guadalajara and took a submarine ride in Aruba. I did not like Jamaica. Nevertheless, we visited them all and saw their sights. However the canal beats everything, it was an engineering feat for its time.

The last cruise was a fifteen-day land-sea tour of Alaska in 2010. We flew into Fairbanks for two days, went gold panning, took a riverboat cruise, and visited Santa at the North Pole. Loved Fairbanks, but too cold in the winter, can drop to 150 below. Then we took the Alaskan Rail to Denali

National Park and spent a night there. We took a bus tour of the Park. Then the train to McKinley for a night. We were blessed we got pictures of the mountain without clouds. The last leg of the train ride was to Anchorage, there we caught a bus to the Kenai Peninsula, stayed two nights there, did some gold panning and river rafting. The bus then took us to the cruise ship through Whittier and this impressive tunnel.

The cruise took us to Vancouver, Canada through the inside passage. However, on the second day at sea, Cody was running a 108 fever and had to be quarantined. He had caught a bad flu. We both were put on Tama-flu medication. That part sucked as your insurance does not work at sea. Thank goodness had enough room on a credit card. The medicine actually worked and by the end of the trip. He was doing fine.

+++

However, eventually, we could not afford to cruise anymore with all the medical bills. We refinanced our house to help pay for a good bulk of the bills. I worked at Nevada Legislation for two sessions. Then, did taxes for four years. In the off-season I work for the Reno Aces Baseball Team, they are a farm team for the Arizona Diamondbacks. I had been there since 2010, Cody was hired 2012. We both love baseball. I love the people, Cody loves the children. Now, I am an author or I should say attempt to be a good writer, but it does not pay much.

It costs over $1000 for each trip to Denver, just for him. If I went, there was at least another $500. Cody makes the trip to Denver at least four times a year and has since 2006. That did not count the two surgeries and infusion treatments. In addition, I had to have knee surgery on both my knees, one replacement, and one repaired. Needless to say, money has become very tight, so we still work. Old age sucks, the only good about the golden years is more time with the grandkids.

Old age is cruel. The sad part is we are not that old. Over the last eleven years, Cody has been in and out of the hospital with a lung virus, lung transplant recipients present an increased risk for severe complications associated with respiratory infections. He has had eye surgery for cataracts due to the medication he has to take. The medication also makes his teeth break or brittle. They check his kidney function as they can be affected by the medicine also. Cody has to watch his skin for cancer, has had two minor surgeries so far, both were cancerous.

"**What is a cataract?**

A cataract is an eye disease in which the normally clear lens of the eye becomes cloudy or opaque, causing a decrease in vision. The lens focuses light onto the back of the eye (the retina), so images appear clear and without distortion. The clouding of this lens during cataract formation distorts vision. Cataracts are usually a very gradual process of normal aging, but can occasionally develop rapidly. They commonly affect both eyes, but it is not uncommon for a cataract in one eye to advance more rapidly. Cataracts are very common, especially among the elderly.

Precisely why cataracts occur is unknown. However, most cataracts appear to be caused by changes in the protein structures within the lens that occur over many years and cause the lens to become cloudy. Rarely, cataracts can present at birth or in early childhood as a result of hereditary enzyme defects, another genetic disease, or systemic congenital infections. Severe trauma to the eye, eye surgery, or intraocular inflammation can also cause cataracts to develop more rapidly. Other factors that may lead to the development of cataracts at an earlier age include excessive ultraviolet light exposure, exposure to ionizing radiation, diabetes, smoking, or the use of certain medications, such as oral, topical, or inhaled steroids. Other medications that may be associated with cataracts include the long-term use of statins and phenothiazines.

The total number of people who have cataracts is estimated to increase to 30.1 million by 2020. When people develop cataracts, they begin to have difficulty doing activities they enjoy. Some of the most common complaints include difficulty driving at night, reading, or traveling. These are all activities for which clear vision is essential.

What are the symptoms and signs of cataracts?

Cataract development is like looking through a dirty windshield of a car or smearing grease over the lens of a camera. Cataracts may cause a variety of complaints and visual changes, including blurred vision, difficulty with glare (often with bright sun or automobile headlights while driving at night), dull color vision, increased nearsightedness accompanied by frequent changes in eyeglass prescription, and occasionally, double vision in one eye. A change in glasses may initially help once vision begins to change from a cataract. However, as the cataract continues to become denser, vision also becomes cloudier, and stronger glasses or contact lenses will no longer improve sight.

Cataracts typically develop gradually and are usually not painful or associated with any eye redness or other symptoms unless they become extremely advanced. Rapid and/or painful changes in vision raise suspicion for other eye diseases and should be evaluated by an eye-care professional.

Eye-care professionals may mention during a routine eye exam that you have early cataract development even if you are not yet experiencing visual symptoms. Although your doctor will be able to tell when you first begin to develop cataracts, you will generally be the first person to notice changes in your vision that may require cataract surgery. Clouding of the lens may start to be seen at any age, but it is uncommon before the age of 40. However, a large majority of people will not begin to have symptoms from their cataracts until many years after they begin to develop. Cataracts can be safely observed without treatment until you notice changes in your vision.

Surgery is recommended for most individuals who have significant vision loss and are symptomatic secondary to cataract. Sometimes after trauma to the eye or previous eye surgery, a cataract may make it difficult for your eye-care professional to see the retina at the back of the eye. In these cases, it may still be appropriate to remove the cataract so that further retinal or optic nerve evaluation and treatment can occur. The mode of surgery can be tailored to individuals based on coexisting medical problems. Cataract surgery is generally performed with minimal sedation and typically takes less than 30 minutes. Therefore the surgery does not put significant strain on the heart or the lungs". (Internet MD)

Mainly all of his illnesses are caused by the medication he takes. Cody takes around 23 pills a day plus his two inhalers. Cost out of our pocket last year was about $33,500 for travel and medication. The cure is killing him more ways than one, but it is worth it. There is no price for life. I tell him every time his feet hit the floor, he has cheated death again.

One of the other things you need to watch is bone density. The medication can affect teeth and bones; here is a little information on those items.

A bone density test determines if you have osteoporosis — a disease that causes bones to become more fragile and more likely to break.

In the past, osteoporosis could be detected only after you broke a bone. By that time, however, your bones could be quite weak. A bone density test enhances the accuracy of calculating your risk of breaking bones.

A bone density test uses X-rays to measure how many grams of calcium and other bone minerals are packed into a segment of bone. The bones that are most commonly tested are in the spine, hip and forearm.

Doctors use bone density testing to:

Identify decreases in bone density before you break a bone

Determine your risk of broken bones (fractures)

Confirm a diagnosis of osteoporosis

Monitor osteoporosis treatment

The higher your bone mineral content, the denser your bones are. And the denser your bones, the stronger they generally are and the less likely they are to break.

Bone density tests differ from bone scans. Bone scans

require an injection beforehand and are usually used to detect fractures, cancer, infections and other abnormalities in the bone.

Although osteoporosis is more common in older women, men also can develop the condition. Regardless of your sex or age, your doctor may recommend a bone density test if you've:

Lost height. People who have lost at least 1.6 inches (4 centimeters) in height may have compression fractures in their spines, for which osteoporosis is one of the leading causes.

Fractured a bone. Fragility fractures occur when a bone becomes so fragile that it breaks much more easily than expected. Fragility fractures can sometimes be caused by a strong cough or sneeze.

Taken certain drugs. Long-term use of steroid medications, such as prednisone, interferes with the bone-rebuilding process — which can lead to osteoporosis.

Received a transplant. People who have received an organ or bone marrow transplant are at higher risk of osteoporosis, partly because anti-rejection drugs also interfere with the bone-rebuilding process.

Teeth: Because saliva helps protect the teeth from decay, transplant patients are at greater risk for tooth decay. Decreased saliva secretion can combine with reduced immunity from the transplant, GVHD of the mouth and immunosuppressive medications to increase the risks of oral infections and oral cancer. Infection in the mouth is most often caused by yeast

All transplant patients should be diligent about daily brushing and flossing. Patients who suffer from dry mouth should follow a program of daily brush-on prescription-strength fluoride gel or other specific treatments to reduce the risk of tooth decay. Routine dental examinations, including X-rays as needed, are important to identify and assess any problems. Decay-associated with mouth dryness can be very aggressive and can cause severe damage. This problem can be reduced or prevented by proper brushing and flossing and daily treatment with prescription-strength fluoride (1.1 percent neutral sodium fluoride).

Patients who are taking immunosuppressive medications and patients with chronic GVHD need effective oral care to prevent inflammation of the gums (gingivitis), periodontal disease and other dental infections. These infections can potentially spread to cause systemic problems and can make GVHD worse.

Therefore, those are some of the hurdles we have to climb, but Cody is doing it.

+++

Last December 2014, Cody turned 65 and had to go

under Medicare plus a bunch of supplemental insurance policies at the cost of $3780 for the year. He still fell into the donut hole on medicine. So right off the top for drugs only, it was over $10,000 a year out of our pocket. This does not include the trips Denver or hospital stays.

"Here is a quick overview of the Donut Hole or Coverage Gap.

According to Medicare (or the Centers for Medicare and Medicaid Services, CMS), Standard or Model Medicare Part D prescription plan, the Donut Hole phase of your Medicare Part D coverage begins when your total retail drug costs reach $3310. (In past coverage years, some Medicare Part D plans have implemented a different Initial Coverage Limit and have begun the Donut Hole phase a little earlier - perhaps at a total retail drug spending of $1,800.)

Please note, this $3310 is the total retail cost of the covered medications, not what you personally spend at the pharmacy. As a Medicare Part D beneficiary, you will pay only a portion of the $3310 and your Part D plan pays a portion. Your total retail cost of prescription medications is calculated from your Medicare Part D plan's negotiated retail drug price - and every Medicare Part D plan can have a different negotiated retail drug price. So it is possible that you may reach the Donut Hole a little earlier or later than someone else who uses the exact same prescription medications, but this other person has enrolled in a prescription drug plan from another Medicare Part D plan provider.

"As a note, in the CMS model Medicare Part D plan, a beneficiary; like yourself, pays the first $360 dollars as an initial deductible and then is responsible for paying 25% of the next $2950, for a total out of pocket medication costs (or true out-of-pocket costs —— TrOOP) of $1097.5 (excluding your monthly plan premiums)." Again, following the CMS standard model Medicare Part D plan, when you reach the Donut Hole, your Medicare Part D plan will have paid the difference between the negotiated retail cost of all your drug purchases and you're out of pocket cost or $2212.5.

However, most people say that you enter the Donut Hole phase of your Medicare Part D plan at the end of your Initial Coverage Phase or when you reach your Medicare Part D plan's Initial Coverage Limit (again, around $3310).

With changes in the Medicare law, a $250 Donut Hole Rebate program was implemented in 2010. Anyone who reached the 2010 Donut Hole was automatically mailed a check for $250. Click here to read some frequently asked questions about the 2010 Donut Hole Rebate.

The 2011 Donut Hole marked the beginning of an effort at closing the Donut Hole. In 2011, anyone reaching the Donut Hole received a 50% discount on brand-name formulary drugs and a 7% discount on all generic formulary medications.

In 2016, anyone reaching the Donut Hole will receive a 55% discount on brand-name formulary drugs and a 42% discount on all generic formulary medications. So for your brand-name drug purchases, you will pay only 45% of the retail cost, but receive 95% credit toward meeting your Donut Hole exit point or TrOOP. For generic drug purchases, you pay 58% of the retail cost and receive the same 58% credit toward TrOOP.

You will stay in the Donut Hole until your TrOOP (True Out-of-Pocket) costs reach $4850". *Medicare rules.*

The bad thing about Medicare and all your supplements is the Donut Hole. We roughly paid out $10,000 the first year for medicine. We cannot maintain that expense, but I cannot let Cody die either. Therefore, even though we have retired, we work to pay medical expenses. Because of our pensions, which are not that much, we still make too much for any help from the Veterans Affairs.

At one point in time, Cody was in acute rejection. He also had bouts of pneumonia. Since 2008 until now, he had had four episodes. The last bout being in January 2017.

"**Acute Rejection:**

Around 60 percent of lung transplant recipients will experience an episode of acute rejection within the first year. Acute rejection is diagnosed by bronchoscopy results, a chest x-ray, and a drop in your Fev1 of greater than 10 percent. Your transplant team will tell you symptoms to look for that may indicate acute rejection. Treatment for acute rejection includes a high dose of corticosteroids. Usually, this consists of three daily doses of intravenous Solu-Medrol, which may be done in a hospital setting or at home, depending on how you feel and your doctor's preference. It is usually followed by a prednisone taper over the next few weeks until you are back down to your baseline dose. Follow-up bronchoscopies may be done to determine whether the rejection is gone.

Unfortunately for some, treatment with corticosteroids may not rid your lungs of acute rejection. Other therapies that can be used if steroids do not help are cytolytic therapy such as rabbit anti-thymocyte globulin (RATG) or horse anti-thymocyte globulin. These are aggressive treatments designed to deplete your T lymphocytes (which are the cause of most acute rejection episodes) and interfere with their normal function. If you need this therapy, you will be monitored in the hospital for the duration of the therapy (5-7 days). There may be some uncomfortable side effects from this treatment. Your doctor will discuss these with you and will also determine what prophylactic medications you may need to prevent infection following the treatment. Because depleting your T-lymphocytes weaken your immune system even further than your maintenance anti-rejection therapy, you will be at increased risk of infection for weeks to months following treatment.

You will need to take the necessary precautions to avoid exposing yourself to infection. If you are still experiencing acute rejection following steroid treatment and anti-thymocyte globulin therapy, you may receive a drug called Campath (alemtuzumab). Campath is an extremely potent medication that can only be given in a hospital setting. It is given as a one-time dose and can cause many side effects. Prophylactic medications must be given for several months to years after the dose is given, and your immune system will be severely compromised for a long time. You must use extreme infection control following Campath. Your doctor will discuss with you the medications you will be taking, how to avoid infections, and how to identify side effects and symptoms of infection." (Medical MD)

Cody exercises every day and tries to walk at least two miles. His hip now is bothering him. For a while, he had a steroid neck from the prednisone. This medication adds weight to you and morphs the body. The neck has, for now, gone away since his lost fifty pounds. That is an accomplishment in its self when you are on that drug.

"Prednisone is a synthetic corticosteroid drug that is particularly effective as an immunosuppressant drug. It is used to treat certain inflammatory diseases (such as moderate allergic reactions) and (at higher doses) some types of cancer but has significant adverse effects.

Prednisone is used for many different indications including: asthma, COPD, CIDP, rheumatic disorders, allergic disorders, ulcerative colitis and Crohn's disease, adrenocortical insufficiency, hypercalcemia due to cancer, thyroiditis, laryngitis, severe tuberculosis, urticaria (hives), lipid pneumonitis, pericarditis, multiple sclerosis, nephrotic syndrome, lupus, myasthenia gravis, poison oak exposure, Meniere's disease, and as part of a drug regimen to prevent rejection after organ transplant.

Prednisone has also been used in the treatment of migraine headaches and cluster headaches and for a severe aphthous ulcer. Prednisone is used as an antitumor drug. It is important in the treatment of acute lymphoblastic leukemia, non-Hodgkin lymphomas, Hodgkin's lymphoma, multiple myeloma, and other hormone-sensitive tumors, in combination with other anticancer drugs.

Prednisone is also used for the treatment of the Herxheimer reaction, which is common during the treatment of syphilis, and to delay the onset of symptoms of Duchenne muscular dystrophy and also for uveitis. The mechanism for the delay of symptoms is unknown. Because it suppresses the adrenal glands, it is also sometimes used in the treatment of congenital adrenal hyperplasia. Prednisone is also used to treat sarcoidosis.

Prednisone can also be used in the treatment of decompensated heart failure to potentiate renal responsiveness to diuretics, especially in heart failure patients with refractory diuretic resistance with a large dose of loop diuretics. The mechanism is prednisone, as a glucocorticoid, can improve renal responsiveness to atrial natriuretic peptide by increasing the density of natriuretic peptide receptor type A in the renal inner medullary collecting duct, inducing a potent diuresis.

Side effects

Short-term side effects, as with all glucocorticoids, include high blood glucose levels (especially in patients with diabetes mellitus or on other medications that increase blood glucose, such as tacrolimus) and mineralocorticoid effects such as fluid retention.[10] The mineralocorticoid effects of prednisone are minor, which is why it is not used in the management of adrenal insufficiency, unless a more potent mineralocorticoid is administered concomitantly. It can also cause depression or depressive symptoms and anxiety in some individuals.

Long-term side effects include Cushing's syndrome, steroid dementia syndrome, truncal weight gain, osteoporosis, glaucoma and cataracts, type II diabetes mellitus, and depression upon dose reduction or cessation." Information from Wikipedia.

+++

However, Cody may be okay for now, but his genuine personality, never came back, mainly due to Prednisone. As I stated earlier, his glass is half empty instead of half full. His strength and will power to live gave him eleven years. However, I do not think he is happy about it sometimes. He tries to be kind and caring, but it is only temporary, and I am not sure it is for real.

Nonetheless, medicine changes people personality, and I try to keep that in mind. Causes of personality change can be a reaction to an especially traumatic event, which may result in severe depression, and we have been through a major life-changing event.

Nevertheless, it is hard. Life changed for all of us with the transplant. He may think he is the only one, but we live with it each day too. Currently, Cody's chronic rejection is in a partial remission, what this means, is if he gets one more cold, he is back on oxygen and then it could be a downhill slide.

CHRONIC REJECTION:

(Bronchiolitis Obliterans Syndrome) The lungs have the highest rate of rejection compared to all other transplanted solid organs. Therefore, life expectancy is shorter for those who have had lung transplants than for those who have had other solid organ transplants.

The number one reason for this is chronic rejection, or BOS (Bronchiolitis Obliterans Syndrome). BOS is present in approximately 48 percent of recipients within five years of the transplant and in 76 percent of recipients within 10 years. This disease course varies among each and every transplant recipient, and some patients will never develop BOS post-transplant.

Diagnosis of BOS is tricky. It can only be detected 30 percent of the time via biopsy taken during a bronchoscopy. Therefore, diagnosis must usually rely on the absence of any other cause for a declining fev1 and a decrease in your forced expiratory flow (FEF 25-75)(lung air volume). Since BOS is characterized by dense fibrous scar tissue in the small airways of the lungs, air may become trapped in the small airways. A chest CT scan may be ordered to determine if air trapping is present. Risk factors for BOS include, but are not limited to:

Gastro-esophageal reflux disease (GERD).*

Numerous acute rejection episodes.*

Poor compliance with anti-rejection treatment.

Primary lung graft dysfunction (PGD).

Fungal, bacterial, and viral infections.*

BOS can also occur without any risk factors present. Treatments that may be tried if BOS is suspected are:

Changing the dose of your anti-rejection medications.*

Adding additional medications to your immunosuppressant*

regimens, such as Cellcept, Everolimus, Sirolimus, or Azithromycin.

RATG (three to five IV doses).

Campath (single IV dose).

Photopheresis treatments.*

A surgical procedure called a Nissen fundoplication (stomach wrap) if GERD is present.

Unfortunately, there are no proven treatments for BOS. The Lung Transplant Foundation's mission is to fund research into this life-shortening syndrome. Multi-center clinical trials are needed to study the onset, progression and treatment options for BOS adequately. As a patient, you do your part by taking the best care of yourself, being compliant with all medications, and reporting any symptoms to your transplant team." (CU) *Cody has had these illnesses or treatments.

Signs of rejection:

fever;

flu-like symptoms, including chills, dizziness, nausea, general feeling of illness, night sweats;

increased difficulty in breathing;

worsening pulmonary test results;

increased chest pain or tenderness;

increase or decrease in body weight of more than two

kilograms in a 24-hour period.

"Chronic rejection is generally considered irreversible and poorly amenable to treatment—only retransplant generally indicated if feasible—though inhaled cyclosporine is being investigated to delay or prevent chronic rejection of lung transplants."

Here is how they figure FEV1:

In general, lung transplant clinicians rely on the absolute values of FVC, FEV1, and FEF25%-75% rather than the percent predicted values. The primary determinants of lung function (FVC and FEV1) are gender, age, height, and race. In general, men have higher lung function than women and lung function peaks between 20 and 30 years of age. In healthy, nonsmoking adults, lung function decreases slowly with age; on average, there is a 30 milliliter per year decrement in FEV1 even in the absence of environmental pollution. This is due to slowly progressive subclinical age-related emphysema. Height is another major determinant of lung function, and taller individuals have higher FVC and FEV1 measurements. Race is the last variable that affects lung function as individuals of different races may have a different trunk to height ratios.

+++

After lung transplantation, there are numerous factors that influence peak lung function. Obviously, bilateral lung recipients will have a higher lung function than single lung recipients. But, there are important donor-related factors that influence lung function. Donor height is the most influential variable; recipients of lungs from taller donors will generally have a higher peak lung function. Donor height is an important factor in donor selection for an individual recipient. Obviously, recipient height will influence this selection. In addition, the recipient's underlying lung disease will determine his or her chest cavity size. For example, emphysema, cystic fibrosis, and obstructive lung diseases, in general, are associated with hyperinflation of the lungs as a result of trapped gas at the end of exhalation. Over time, this results in hyperinflation of the chest cavity size. In contrast, pulmonary fibrosis progressively reduces lung volumes, and there is a concomitant decrease in chest cavity size over time. As a result, patients with obstructive lung diseases can generally accept lungs from donors who are taller than they are while those with restrictive lung diseases such as pulmonary fibrosis generally have to have donors who are shorter than they are, and this will influence peak lung function after transplant. For example, some patients with emphysema may have peak FVC and FEV1 measurements over 100%, and sometimes over 130%, of their predicted values after transplantation, while some patients with pulmonary fibrosis may have peak FVC and FEV1 measurements 70-75% of their predicted values.

Nonetheless, although their lung function is lower than predicted, these patients usually have no functional or clinically significant limitations.

In addition, complications early after transplantation may affect peak lung function. Recipients who develop severe primary graft dysfunction (PGD) tend to have lower maximal lung function after transplantation because of resultant scarring. Similarly, recipients who develop severe pneumonia in the early period after transplantation typically have reduced peak lung function. For these reasons, lung transplant clinicians rely primarily on the absolute values of FVC and FEV1 rather than the percent predicted values, and track these longitudinally. The best lung function is defined as the average of the two highest measurements after transplantation, and subsequent changes in lung function are compared to this average. In summary, there are multiple determinants of maximal lung function after transplantation, and different patients will likely have different peak lung function because of donor-related factors and early post-operative complications. (CU)

Chapter Twelve – Today

November 2015, Cody went to the hospital with Atrial fibrillation, they think it was caused due to a reaction to his flu shot and his transplant medicine.

"Atrial fibrillation (A-tre-al fi-bri-LA-shun), or AF, is the most common type of arrhythmia (ah-RITH-me-ah). An arrhythmia is a problem with the rate or rhythm of the heartbeat. During an arrhythmia, the heart can beat too fast, too slow, or with an irregular rhythm.

AF occurs if rapid, disorganized electrical signals cause the heart's two upper chambers—called the atria (AY-tree-uh)—to fibrillate. The term "fibrillate" means to contract very fast and irregularly.

In AF, blood pools in the atria. It is not pumped completely into the heart's two lower chambers, called the ventricles (VEN-trih-kuls). As a result, the heart's upper and lower chambers do not work together as they should.

People who have AF may not feel symptoms. However, even when AF is not noticed, it can increase the risk of stroke. In some people, AF can cause chest pain or heart failure, especially if the heart rhythm is very rapid.

AF may rarely happen or every now and then, or it may become an ongoing or long-term heart problem that lasts for years." (Wikipedia)

Cody also had a c-scan with contrast agents to check for blood clots as they appeared in his x-rays.

> "CT contrast agents, sometimes referred to as "dyes," are used to highlight specific areas so that the organs, blood vessels, or tissues are more visible. By increasing the visibility of all surfaces of the organ or tissue being studied, they can help the radiologist determine the presence and extent of disease or injury". (Dictionary)

Therefore, he spent Saturday night and most of Sunday in the hospital. Now he will have stress tests to see if something else is going on. The hospital changed some of his medication and Denver now wants blood work to make sure the Prograf level stay the same.

"Prograf:

Is a medicine that slows down the body's immune system. For this reason, it works as an anti-rejection medication. Prograf helps patients who have had a liver/kidney or lung transplant protect their new organ and prevent it from being rejected by the body. This medicine can cause the amount of potassium in your blood stream to increase. For this reason, you should avoid large amounts of foods that have a high potassium content, for example, dried fruit, bananas, tomatoes, and a low sodium salt, while you are taking this medicine, also avoid potassium supplements. You can get a bad reaction from eating these foods. We had been warned about grapefruit juice, as it increases the amount of Prograf in the blood stream." (Medical MD)

Therefore, he will have blood work every 30 days to watch the Prograf levels. They adjusted his blood pressure medicine as he has pulmonary hypertension.

"Pulmonary hypertension:

Is a type of high blood pressure that affects the arteries in the lungs and the right side of your heart.

Pulmonary hypertension begins when tiny arteries in your lungs, called pulmonary arteries, and capillaries become narrowed, blocked, or destroyed. This makes it harder for blood to flow through your lungs and raises the pressure within your lungs' arteries. As the pressure builds, your heart's lower right chamber (right ventricle) must work harder to pump blood through your lungs, eventually causing your heart muscle to weaken and eventually fail.

Pulmonary hypertension is a serious illness that becomes progressively worse and is sometimes fatal. Although pulmonary hypertension is not curable, treatments are available that can help lessen symptoms and improve your quality of life". (CU)

After Cody seeing his primary doctor, they scheduled him to see a heart doctor and have a bunch of stress tests.

Below is what is involved.

"**A cardiac stress test** (or cardiac diagnostic test) is a cardiological test that measures a heart's ability to respond to external stress in a controlled clinical environment. The stress response is induced by exercise or by drug stimulation.

Cardiac stress tests compare the coronary circulation while the patient is at rest with the same patient's circulation during maximum physical exertion, showing any abnormal blood flow to the myocardium (heart muscle tissue). The results can be interpreted as a reflection on the general physical condition of the test patient. This test can be used to diagnose coronary artery disease (also known as ischemic heart disease), and for patient prognosis after a myocardial infarction (heart attack).

The cardiac stress test is done with heart stimulation, either by exercise on a treadmill, pedaling a stationary exercise bicycle ergometer or with intravenous pharmacological stimulation, with the patient connected to an electrocardiogram (ECG). People who cannot use their legs may exercise with a bicycle-like crank that they turn with their arms.

The level of mechanical stress is progressively increased by adjusting the difficulty (steepness of the slope) and speed. The test administrator or attending physician examines the symptoms and blood pressure response. With the use of ECG, the test is most commonly called a cardiac stress test, but is known by other names, such as exercise testing, stress testing treadmills, exercise tolerance test, stress test, or stress test ECG.

A stress test may also use an echocardiogram (ultrasonic imaging of the heart), or a nuclear stress test (in which a radioisotope dye is injected into the bloodstream)."

On top of the stress test, he have more blood work so they can adjusted his medicine, which now Denver will have to adjust his transplant medicine. It is a snowball reaction.

+++

On a positive side, Cody does attend pre-transplant meetings, answering questions from patients waiting or their families. The doctors can tell patients about the transplant, but they want to know from Cody how it will feel. I believe he was predestined to have an illness that led to his transplant so he can help other patients and families. We both hope to help raise awareness of the importance of organ donation.

Even if the patient only gets one more year of life, it is better than the alternative. In Cody's case, he has beaten the odds with eleven years out. We are hoping for a whole bunch more.

Cody and the physicians all agree that patients need to believe in themselves and adopt a mindset that failure is not an option. Attitude can go a long way toward helping you, both during the time you're waiting for a transplant and during recovery from transplant. Cody is living proof that being dedicated to your own health can be a difference maker. I also tease him about having nine lives.

Chapter Thirteen - Thankful for the Donor

Here is some information you may want to include in your letter to the donor's family:

Your first name only

The state where you live

Recognize the donor family and thank them for their gift

How long you waited for a transplant and how the wait affected you and your family

How the transplant has improved your health and changed your life

What has happened in your life since the transplant?

Mention if you are married, have children, grandchildren, etc.

State your hobbies or interests

What information should not be included?

Do not include your address, city or phone number

Do not include the name or location of the hospital where your transplant surgery was performed, nor the names of your transplant health care providers

Use caution when including religious comments, as you do not know the religion of the donor's family

How can I send the letter to my donor's family?

After you write a letter to the donor's family, place it an unsealed envelope (the correspondence is reviewed for confidentiality) and include a separate sheet of paper with your full name and date of transplant. Send this information in a separate envelope to:

Lung Transplant Coordinator

The Cleveland Clinic Foundation

9500 Euclid Avenue, A110

Cleveland, OH 44195

After receiving your correspondence, the transplant coordinator forwards it to LifeBanc, northeastern Ohio's organ procurement agency. LifeBanc will notify the donor's family that there is correspondence from the recipient."

"You may or may not hear from your donor's family. Some donor families may feel that writing about their loved one and their decision to donate helps them with their grieving. Others choose not to write to the organ recipient.

If the donor's family wants to respond, they will send a letter to LifeBanc. LifeBanc will forward the correspondence to your transplant coordinator, who will forward the response to you.

Many years ago, we were able to write to the family of the man who gave Cody his lungs. We were so thankful. We had to wait a year to write to the family. They did respond giving us his name, which was Nate; that is why this story is a gift from Nate. He was 21; they did not say how he died and apparently they did not want to stay in contact with us.

We do not know what happened to cause such a young man to die, but we are so thankful to his family for his lungs, and we are aware several other families are also thankful who received his liver and kidneys. We understood no one received his heart, so you can only assume he had a heart attack of some sort.

It is an emotional gift, knowing someone died so you could live, and we will never be able to thank them enough.

Since Cody received his lungs, there has been so much more improvement in the lung transplant field. The only concern is a lack of trained doctors and hospitals to treat the lung recipients. When Cody gets sick, it is a major problem to get him the help that is needed in Nevada. Therefore, we must go back to Denver to get proper care.

The greatest gift of love that anyone could ever give is the gift of life. When that gift is given, a life lives on. The spirit of Cody's donor is in him, and we only wish we knew more about him. Cody did thank the family personally and learn a little about Nate. Thank you to all the organ donors out there! You are all heroes!

Chapter Fourteen – Information: The effects of Lung Failure; Stories from Transplant Patients; and Other medical information.

Chronic Rejection:

Because the cause of BO is unknown, in 1993 the International Society for Heart and Lung Transplantation coined the term "bronchiolitis obliterans syndrome" (BOS) to describe deterioration of lung function for which there is no other identifiable cause. Patients have BOS if there is a 20% reduction in their FEV1 (forced expired volume in 1 second) from their previously established baseline.

Unfortunately, chronic rejection is a difficult condition to treat. There are several medications shown to arrest or stabilize the progression of the condition. Radiation therapy has also shown to be effective. New medications currently in clinical trials hold promise for improvements in future treatment and prevention of chronic rejection.

"Chronic rejection is less well defined than either hyperacute or acute rejection. It is probably caused by multiple factors: antibodies as well as lymphocytes. The definitive diagnosis of chronic rejection is again generally made by biopsy of the organ in question. The heart is an exception to this generalization: chronic rejection in heart grafts is felt to be manifest by accelerated graft atherosclerosis. In other words, the transplanted heart rapidly develops "hardening of the arteries." Kidneys with chronic rejection have fibrosis (scarring) and damage to the microscopic blood vessels in the substance of the kidney. Livers with chronic rejection have a decreased number of bile ducts on biopsy. This is referred to as the "vanishing bile duct syndrome." Transplanted lungs with chronic rejection are said to have "bronchiolitis obliterans" a scarring problem in the substance of the lung."

To date, most research has focused on graft survival for the first three years. It is not that we, the physicians involved with transplantation, don't care about long-term results. The long term problem is simply tough to tackle. Animal models exist, but they do not perfectly reflect what goes on in humans. Most studies on people that look at long-term outcome are not well "controlled," so their conclusions are nebulous. To be "controlled" a study needs to have two groups of patients, one that received a particular treatment and one that didn't. The best kind of controlled study is prospective and randomized, meaning the decision as to which treatment the patient has been decided before the treatment begins in a random fashion. This eliminates many biases that otherwise appear. These studies take very long time periods, are extremely difficult and labor intensive and requires large numbers of patients to look at long term results. More typically, studies use "historical controls" meaning that one group, say patients transplanted from 1987 to 1990 is compared to another group of patients transplanted at a different time point, like 1984 to 1986. The problem with such studies is that so many things changed between the two groups. Techniques change better perfusion solutions for the organs, quicker, more accurate methods of measuring blood levels of cyclosporine ("Sandimmune").

New agents, like FK506 (tacrolimus or "Prograf") are introduced and other agents are removed from the market. Understanding of common infections in transplant patients improves; this improves overall results even though the improvement wasn't exactly related to what immunosuppression they received. The studies, therefore, get muddled over the years. To look at ten-year results today, we have to look at transplants that were done in 1985 when techniques were significantly different in many ways from the way we do things now. So the bottom line is that much of what we do today is not firmly based on actual evidence that it is the one best treatment. He explains why different transplant centers do different things: their particular experience has been based on the specific patient population.

Fortunately, much work is currently being done on

chronic rejection, both in the lab and clinically. Some new agents not yet in use clinically look to be particularly effective at combating chronic rejection. As these new drugs appear long-term graft survival will hopefully increase. In many situations, the current standard treatment for chronic rejection is retransplantation. This approach is not satisfactory, however, because it makes the existing organ shortage worse, and retransplantation is more difficult from a surgical perspective."

What happens when the lungs fail, whether after one year or twenty years?

"Pulmonary complications have been observed in 40 to 60% of patients after allogeneic hematopoietic cell transplant (HCT). Complications may be infectious or noninfectious such as pulmonary edema, diffuse alveolar hemorrhage, idiopathic pneumonia syndrome, or bronchiolitis obliterans (1). Pulmonary complications have been associated with decreased post-transplant pulmonary function, including reductions in forced expiratory volume in 1 second (FEV1), forced vital capacity (FVC), total lung capacity (TLC), or a decrease in diffusion capacity for carbon monoxide (DLCO). Many factors may affect pulmonary function after HCT including the underlying disease process, conditioning regimen, infections, and the development of acute or chronic graft-versus-host disease (GVHD).

While previous studies have characterized the clinical scenarios associated with decreased lung function after transplantation, most cohorts were small and primarily descriptive. One large study published in 1995 reported a two-fold increase in the risk of non-relapse mortality associated with the development of restrictive lung defects after transplantation, but restrictive lung disease was not associated with developing chronic GVHD. Despite the limitations of these studies, they suggest that post-transplant lung function changes may be useful for assessing a patient's risk for various transplant-related outcomes, such as the development of GVHD and mortality.

In 2005, the National Institutes of Health (NIH) Consensus Development Project on Criteria for Clinical Trials in Chronic GVHD proposed new recommendations to improve the diagnosis and grading of chronic GVHD. Calculation of a lung function score (LFS) was recommended to grade the extent of lung function compromise after a diagnosis of chronic GVHD had been established (13). However, the LFS is based on an algorithm developed originally for grading pre-transplant lung function. The relationship between lung function, mortality, and chronic GVHD has not been rigorously analyzed using post-transplant lung function. To address this gap, we conducted a retrospective cohort study of patients who underwent HCT during a 12-year period to examine the relationship of post-transplant pulmonary function testing (PFT) with 5-year mortality. We further evaluated the relationship between post-transplant lung function and the development of chronic GVHD according to NIH criteria.

All patients who had HCT at Fred Hutchinson Cancer Research Center (FHCRC) or Seattle Cancer Care Alliance between January 1992 and December 2004 were potentially eligible. Patients who were younger than 15 years, died before pulmonary function testing (PFT) or did not have PFT were excluded (Figure 1). All clinical data except for chronic GVHD status were prospectively collected and retrospectively analyzed. Chronic GVHD data according to NIH criteria was collected retrospectively. The patient's underlying disease state was categorized as low, intermediate, or high risk as previously described (14, 15). Donor match status was determined according to donor–recipient HLA compatibility. Stem cell sources were classified as bone marrow, peripheral blood stem cell, or a combination of both. Conditioning regimens were classified as nonmyeloablative or myeloablative. Subjects in the myeloablative group were subdivided as receiving either a total body irradiation (TBI) or non–TBI based regimen. Acute GVHD was graded based on stages of organ involvement using standard criteria (15, 16). Ethnicity was self-reported. Using clinical records, all patients were followed from transplant until death or January 04, 2008. This study was approved by the institutional review board at FHCRC.

Lung Function Testing

All pulmonary function testing was performed at our Center, according to American Thoracic Society guidelines (17), using the Sensormedics 2100 (Sensormedics Co., Yorba Linda, CA) from January 1992 to August 1999, and the Sensormedics V-Max 22 with Auto box 6200 from September 1999 to December 2004. Published equations for adults were used to determine predicted values of FEV1, FVC, TLC and DLCO (18). All DLCO measurements were corrected for the hemoglobin measurement obtained closest to the time the diffusion capacity was measured (19). All PFT values, except FEV1/FVC ratio, were expressed as a percentage of predicted values and assessed categorically. PFT categories were defined as normal (≥80%), mildly abnormal (70–79%), moderately abnormal (60–69%) or severely abnormal (<60%). Per NIH recommendations, the lung function score (LFS) was calculated according to the day 80 FEV1 and DLCO, each of which was mapped to a category as follows: (≥80% = 1, 70–79% = 2, 60–69% = 3, 50–59% = 4, 40–49% = 5, and <40% = 6) (13, 14). Scores for FEV1 and DLCO were then summed, and categorized 0 to 3 as defined by NIH recommendations [LFS score 2 = category 0 (normal); LFS score 3–5 = category 1 (mildly abnormal); LFS score 6–9 = category 2 (moderately abnormal); or LFS score 10–12 = category 3 (severely abnormal)].

Chronic GVHD analysis

Chronic GVHD data was available for a subset of the cohort. As part of a separate study, 2602 patients with a history of a myeloablative transplant between 1992 and 2005 had undergone a retrospective chart review to establish a diagnosis of chronic GVHD according to current NIH guidelines (13). Patients who had undergone this chronic GVHD assessment and who had day 80 PFT were eligible for the chronic GVHD analysis.

Statistical Methods

All analyses were performed using STATA 10.0 (StataCorp, College Station, TX). Two-tailed P-values <0.05 were considered statistically significant. All data were analyzed as categorical variables except age (continuous). Robust standard errors using a sandwich estimator were calculated for all analyses. Models were compared using Harrell's C-statistic. The C-statistic is the proportion of predicted outcomes and observed results that are concordant. The primary exposure was LFS category and primary outcome 5-year non-relapse mortality.

Secondary exposures were individual PFT parameters. Cox proportional hazards models were used to evaluate the association between non-relapse mortality and lung function. All multivariable analyses were adjusted for covariates that may be associated with lung function, chronic GVHD, and mortality. These variables included age, sex, disease risk, conditioning regimen, HLA status, acute **GVHD,** and prior CMV infection in the donor and patient as determined by serological testing. Patients who had recurrent malignancy before PFT were excluded from hazard models (n=61). Survival was censored at 5 years from transplant or at a diagnosis of recurrent malignancy.

A secondary analysis used development of chronic GVHD within one year of PFT as the primary outcome. LFS category was the primary exposure. Patients who had recurrent malignancy before PFT were excluded. Those with a diagnosis of chronic GVHD prior to, or within one week of PFT were also excluded. Survival was censored at death, the onset of recurrent malignancy, or one year following PFT.

Results

Between January 1992 and December 2004, 3548 patients underwent HCT. After excluding subjects < 15 years of age (12%), those who died before day 80 PFT (19%) and those without day 80 PFT data (8%), 2158 patients were included in the analysis (Figure 1). Patients were followed for a median (IQR) of 1312 (251–1826) days. The median (IQR) time from transplant until the day 80 PFT was 78 (76–83) days.

This summarizes the clinical characteristics of the full cohort and the cohort who underwent an analysis for GVHD. The majority of patients had normal lung function. The mean FEV1, FVC, and TLC were 88 ± 15%, 93 ± 16%, and 97 ± 15% respectively. The mean DLCO was 81 ± 18% and was less than 80% in 49% of patients. Twelve percent of patients met criteria for obstructive lung disease, defined by an FEV1/FVC ratio < 0.7. Of patients with obstructive lung disease, the FEV1 was ≥ 80% in nearly one-half of patients and < 60% in 12% of patients. Twelve percent of patients had restrictive lung disease, defined as TLC < 80% predicted. Of patients with restrictive lung disease, the FEV1 was ≥ 80% in 16% and < 60% in 21% of patients. Forty-two percent of patients were in LFS category 0. These patients had both an FEV1 and DLCO ≥ 80% predicted. Forty-two percent of patients were in LFS category 1. These patients had either a mildly abnormal FEV1, DLCO, or both. Nine percent of patients were in LFS Category 2, and 1% were in Category 3. Patients in LFS category 3 had severely abnormal lung function representing both an FEV1 and DLCO no higher than 60% predicted. Five-year all-cause mortality was 40%, and 5-year non-relapse mortality was 20%. Five-year relapse was 28%.

Seventy-two patients (4%) were diagnosed with chronic GVHD before or within one week of PFT and were excluded from the chronic GVHD analysis. The remaining 1650 patients evaluated for chronic GVHD were similar to the entire cohort except a slightly higher percentage had a bone marrow stem cell source (69%), and very few (<1%) had a non-myeloablative conditioning regimen. The distribution of day 80 PFTs for this cohort is summarized in Table 3. Overall 846 (51%) developed chronic GVHD, and 726 were diagnosed within 1 year of PFT.

Lung function and mortality

Diminished lung function at day 80 post-transplant was associated with an increased risk of non-relapse mortality at five years as measured by lung function score. Patients in LFS category 1 had a nearly 50% increased risk of death. This risk increased to more than 3-fold for patients in category 2 and nearly 8-fold in category 3. All hazard ratio estimates were statistically significant. The trend of increased mortality with increasing LFS category was statistically significant (p < 0.0005). After adjustment for age, sex, disease risk, conditioning regimen, HLA compatibility, acute GVHD, donor and patient CMV status, and pre-HCT lung function, hazard ratios were largely unchanged [category 1 HR 1.37 (1.08–1.75); category 2 HR 3.02 (2.11–4.33); category 3 HR 8.56 (4.54–16.14)]. The trend remained statistically significant (p<0.0005).

There was also a stepwise increase in the risk of

mortality associated with individual PFT parameters. Compared to a normal FEV1, a mildly decreased FEV1 was associated with a 76% increased risk of mortality [HR 1.76 (1.38–2.24)]. The HR increased to 2.33 (1.68–3.25), and 5.79 (4.28–7.85) for a moderate and severely decreased FEV1, respectively. A similar increase in HR was seen for FVC. Although the relationship was not as distinct for TLC categories, hazard ratio estimates for each category were also significantly increased. For DLCO, this association was only significant for categories 2 and 3 [category 2 HR 2.04 (1.57–2.66); category 3 HR 1.96–3.43)]. Similar to LFS, the trend towards increased mortality with decreasing pulmonary function was statistically significant for all PFT parameters (p<0.0005). Figure 2 demonstrates the 5-year cumulative incidence of non-relapse mortality as a function of PFT parameters and LFS categories. After adjustment, hazard ratio estimates were largely unchanged and remained statistically significant for all PFT parameters except DLCO category 1. There was no significant relationship between mortality and FEV1/FVC ratio [HR 1.11 (0.92–1.36)].

Although previous studies have evaluated lung function after HCT (2–11), few studies have critically examined whether lung function observed within the first 100 days after transplantation is associated with long-term clinical events. Instead, several previous studies have suggested that pulmonary function abnormalities within the first 6 months after transplant may be the result of peritransplant events, may be reversible, and may have no prognostic value (2). Our results show the contrary, indicating that diminished lung function at day 80 following transplant was significantly associated with poor long-term outcomes. Especially, patients with the most severely abnormal lung function, as measured by the LFS, had a nearly 8-fold higher risk of 5-year non-relapse mortality. An increased risk was also seen with individual pulmonary function parameters. Our results also show that early posttransplant pulmonary dysfunction may identify patients at risk of developing chronic GVHD. While this relationship was present for the LFS, the clearest association was with FEV1. These results suggest that diminished lung function posttransplant should not be dismissed as a transient finding. Moreover, routine pulmonary function testing following transplant may identify a group of higher risk patients who need to be followed closely for posttransplant complications and signs of chronic GVHD.

Models using either the LFS or individual PFT parameters performed similarly. These results suggest that individual PFT parameters, especially FEV1, may be as informative as the LFS, making it reasonable to assess spirometry alone for routine monitoring of lung function after HCT. This practice would result in a decrease in cost and increase in accessibility of lung function monitoring and thus increase the likelihood that monitoring will be adopted more widely as standard clinical practice for the management of all HCT patients.

Crawford et al. previously showed that diminished lung function after transplant was associated with late mortality (5). A restrictive lung defect at day 80 or a decrease in TLC of 15% or greater from baseline was associated with a 2-fold increased risk of mortality. FEV1/FVC ratio and DLCO were not significantly associated with mortality. In our study, all PFT parameters except for FEV1/FVC ratio were associated with mortality. Several reasons might explain why our results differ. Crawford et al. classified an abnormal DLCO as < 80%, a threshold that may have been too high to identify patients with clinically significant pulmonary compromise. Our study was larger and divided patients with an abnormal DLCO as mild, moderate, and severe. We did not find a significant association for patients with a mildly abnormal DLCO (70–80%), but an association was present for a DLCO less than 70%. Furthermore, Crawford et al. described a cohort who had HCT before 1990. Posttransplant care has changed significantly since then. Nonmyeloablative conditioning regimens are now frequently used and associated with fewer pulmonary complications (20), and preemptive antifungal and anti-CMV treatment are also more readily available (21). Both changes have improved outcomes after HCT.

Crawford et al. did not detect an association between TLC and chronic GVHD (5). We also did not find an association between TLC and chronic GVHD. Chronic GVHD of the lungs manifests as bronchiolitis obliterans and airflow obstruction, which may explain why FEV1, and not TLC, was associated with the development of chronic GVHD in our study.

Pulmonary dysfunction following HCT has several possible causes. Patients are at increased risk of respiratory infections due to prolonged immunosuppression (1, 21). Chemotherapeutics may have direct toxic effects such as damage to vascular endothelium or alveoli resulting in a decreased DLCO. Chest wall, mediastinal, or total body irradiation may have short and long-term effects on pulmonary function (22). Acute and chronic GVHD have been previously associated with a diminished posttransplant pulmonary function (4, 7, 9). However, previous studies were unable to ascertain whether the diminished pulmonary function was the result of chronic GVHD or was an early marker of chronic GVHD. Additionally, these studies were conducted before NIH consensus definitions. Strengths of our study were ascertainment of the date chronic GVHD was diagnosed, restriction of our analysis to patients without a diagnosis of chronic GVHD at day 80, and the use of current NIH criteria for the diagnosis of chronic GVHD.

Our results should be interpreted with some caution. First, day 80 PFTs were not available for the entire cohort. A post hoc analysis of patients who survived for at least 60 days, and therefore could have had PFT but did not (n=527, 15%), showed that 81% of these patients died. It may be that patients missing PFT carried a higher burden of illness and were either unable to have testing, or providers were reluctant to subject them to testing. If true, this practice would tend to bias our results away from the null hypothesis and strengthen our findings. Second, our single center results might not apply to other centers. In the GVHD analysis, we used current NIH diagnostic criteria in an attempt to minimize this limitation. Third, the diagnosis of chronic GVHD according to NIH criteria was retrospective and subject to misclassification; and some patients may have had undiagnosed chronic GVHD when the pulmonary function was evaluated. Finally, we were unable to determine the cause of non-relapse mortality as patients are routinely discharged from our Center around day 100. Many deaths that occur outside the Seattle region.

In summary, we have shown that decreased pulmonary function after transplant was associated with an increased risk of 5-year non-relapse mortality. Decreased FEV1 was also associated with the development of chronic GVHD within the first year after the day 80 PFT. Pulmonary dysfunction can be graded with the NIH recommended LFS, but a simple assessment of FEV1 can provide similarly useful clinical information. Future studies should focus on validation of our findings and should examine these associations using additional pulmonary function assessments at one year or later following transplant. In the meantime, these data provide evidence supporting the NIH recommendation that pulmonary function should be routinely monitored after HCT. Patients who have significantly abnormal lung function should be followed closely for complications or signs of chronic GVHD.

Information from the US National Library of Medicine."

+++

What this all means is when the lungs fail, Cody goes back on oxygen, then the carbon monoxide builds up in his lungs over time, and he will suffocate. This could take years, in the meantime, other diseases could terminate his life, just like the rest of us. We could all be hit by a car or shot by a terrorist.

Having the transplant even with all the concerns, medication, cost and other illness, it is worth it to get to see your granddaughter graduate from high school or college.

+++

As mentioned earlier, Cody goes to Denver twice to four times a year, when we are in the clinic, I talk to other recipients or their family about what is going on with them. People come from all over the country to Colorado, even from other major clinics. After reading these stories, you will see how important it is to be a donor. Here are some of the stories:

When a doctor suddenly becomes the patient with a life-threatening illness, Mayo Clinic's commitment to high-quality medical care that puts the needs of the patient first takes on a fresh perspective, especially as it relates to the principle of compassionate care, which is a hallmark of Mayo Clinic.

Such was the case when Joseph T, M.D., a 68-year-old pediatric surgeon learned that the wheezing and shortness of breath he was experiencing turned out to be idiopathic pulmonary fibrosis, a potentially life-threatening disease that occurs from unexplained scarring of the lung tissue.

In addition to doing pediatric surgery, Dr. T is a practicing trauma surgeon and surgical intensivist. He is the medical director of the region's only pediatric trauma unit, and, as a retired captain in the Navy Reserve, appreciates the critical importance of maintaining a personal commitment to health and fitness. Dr. T had always lived a healthy lifestyle and, other than some occasional allergy symptoms, never had any significant health issues. But lying dormant in his otherwise healthy body was a disease that was quietly scarring and shutting his lungs down.

"When I saw the CT scan, I could clearly see that both my lungs were pretty much gone," says Dr. Tepas. "My otherwise healthy lifestyle and physical fitness were masking the disease that was silently killing me."

The speed in which Dr. T discovered, and was ultimately diagnosed and treated for his serious illness, was impressive. Dr. T first experienced his symptoms on a trip to Washington, D.C., and figured the inhaler, his doctor prescribed would manage the wheezing and shortness of breath. When it became apparent what he was experiencing was more severe, he underwent a series of tests and discovered his shocking diagnosis – idiopathic pulmonary fibrosis and acute interstitial pneumonia (Hamman-Rich Syndrome, a rare form of rapidly progressive end-stage lung disease). It soon became apparent that he was going to need a double lung transplant if he was going to survive. Given the accelerating deterioration of his lung function, Dr. T was emergently referred to Mayo Clinic for a transplant evaluation. Within 36 hours of arrival, he had received a full assessment of his condition and was immediately put on the UNOS transplant list.

With his condition dire, he was very fortunate to get some good news after only two days on the list – a new pair of lungs from a 24-year-old matching donor had become available. Dr. T was transplanted on July 21, 2014, less than six weeks after he first realized he was seriously ill. He was released from the hospital just two weeks later. "I think that may be a record," says Dr. T. "The fact that I was in good physiological shape was a big factor in helping speed up my immediate post-surgical recovery. The rapidity with which a donor was found was nothing short of miraculous!"

And although he works at a different regional hospital, Dr. T had nothing but praise for Mayo Clinic and its transplant capabilities.

"Mayo does it right, from the procedural training of its staff to their consistent reflection of genuine interest in the patient's well-being," he says. "My care was spectacular across the board, from my surgeon and pulmonary team to the nurses and technicians who took care of me throughout my stay in the hospital. I'm truly appreciative to all of them, not just for the excellent care I received, but for the constant concern and compassion with which it was always provided."

There is an interesting twist to this story relating to the importance of organ donation. Dr. T was the trauma surgeon on call in 1998 when a 17-year-old Jacksonville teenager named Katie Caples was brought to him in critical condition after a motor vehicle crash. Although Katie passed away as a result of her brain injuries, she donated her organs to five different recipients (ages 9 to 62), since she was a registered organ donor. Her father, David Caples, started the Katie Caples Foundation and its annual organ donation awareness and education event, The Katie Ride for Life, in 2005. It is held annually in Amelia Island, Florida, and raises money to educate high school students in Northeast Florida about the importance of organ donation. Mayo Clinic has been a major sponsor and supporter of the event for the past several years.

"In many ways, Katie Caples was the personification of my own daughter, who also happens to be named Katie, who was also a cross country runner, and who went to the same high school," says Dr. T. "I've maintained a relationship with the Caples family since the accident and have participated in several of the Katie Ride events over the years. Mayo Clinic's involvement as a sponsor and active participant in that event is a natural, given its expertise in organ transplantation and interest in spreading the word about the importance of organ donation. Little did I know that someday the same transplant service that works so many miracles on a daily basis would reach out to save the life of the surgeon who had initially tried to save Katie."

Here is another story, this is why it is so important to be a donor.

Sometimes miracles happen when you least expect

them. No one believes that more than Shirley T, whose tale of how she received two new lungs while in a medically induced coma at Mayo Clinic hospital isn't exactly the typical scenario.

The 48-year old, married, mother of two was first diagnosed with Pulmonary Arterial Hypertension (PAH) in March 2012 by her local pulmonologist after undergoing an EKG and experiencing shortness of breath. She was eventually referred to Mayo Clinic for an evaluation and was put on continuous High flow oxygen during treatment for her lung condition.Ms. T re-entered the hospital in October 2012 for an unrelated hysterectomy surgery, and that's when her condition took a dramatic turn for the worse. Her lung (and related heart) problems worsened after the surgery, and she was then put in a medically induced coma once it was determined that she was going to need a double lung transplant and heart surgery in order to survive.

That's when her miracle happened. During the several weeks, she was in a coma at Mayo Clinic hospital, a potential donor became available, "literally down the hallway" and eventually became a perfect match for Ms. T's much needed double lung transplant. When she awoke from her coma, she realized she had been given the gift of life without ever knowing it.

"I didn't know I needed a lung transplant before my hysterectomy surgery and wasn't even on the transplant list at the time," said Ms. T. "I had no idea the situation had become so serious that a double lung transplant was immediately needed to save my life. I was fortunate to have a generous donor in the right place at the right time, and I will forever be grateful for their gift of life."

"Ms. T's situation is truly a miracle scenario where the stars all aligned at the right time and a matching organ was available right down the hall in the same hospital when it was most needed," said Cesar Keller, M.D., the pulmonary and critical care specialist at Mayo Clinic who was responsible for her care. "This is a true success story and an excellent example of how organ donation can help save a life."

Although still not 100% back to normal, Ms. T is feeling better each day and no longer needs to carry supplemental oxygen which makes daily life a bit easier. "I cannot say enough about my doctors at Mayo Clinic who are amazing, I know without a doubt I would not be alive today without their efforts."

And another:

Tevis M has suffered from a chronic lung infection all of his life, a debilitating condition called bronchiectasis that kept him tethered to an oxygen tank and threatened his life.

"It got so that I couldn't do anything at all," he says. "I was on oxygen 24/7. You know those little plastic sticks that have little holes in it that you stir your coffee? Try breathing through that sometimes, and that's what it was like."

But after undergoing a double lung transplant at Ronald Reagan UCLA Medical Center, Tevis is now beginning a new life.

A cardiothoracic surgeon, Dr. A. performed the delicate lung transplant. "In contrast to the other organs, such as kidney and liver where the time is more forgiving, for heart and lung transplantation, every minute that the organ is outside of the body is important," Dr. A. explains.

The first 10 minutes following implantation are the most critical for the new lungs to function. "Throughout our experience and many years of research at UCLA, we have devised an approach that we believe improves the function of the lungs in the long term," Dr. A. says.

Now Tevis is able to do many things that he wasn't able to do before the transplant, and Dr. A. expects there will be an even greater improvement as he becomes accustomed to his new lungs.

"Just to have it done is a miracle," Tevis says. "It's like if you were to take a light switch and turn it off or turn it on, that's the difference of how I feel."

Here is another, these stories are so important, and they are real people.

I just wanted to offer a little history about me and COPD and Lung Transplants. This ought to be pretty boring, so I recommend pressing the <-Backspace key now unless you really have nothing to do :-)

My mother died of emphysema in her early 60's in 1990. My brothers both have lung disease, and my daughter has a little asthma.

I was diagnosed with COPD about 20 years ago. So there is something hereditary going on. My mother and I both smoked cigarettes, but my brothers did not, so they are not as bad off.

A few years ago, I was recommended for LVRS surgery, but at the time it was experimental and had an 80% survival rate, so I opted out. At the time, my FEV1 was about 33%, and I was not yet on oxygen. After a few years, my health degraded to the point where my FEV1 was 11%, I was on 6 liters of O2 at rest and spent much of my time in a wheelchair.

I had stopped working (mainly because of the economy after 9/11. I was a systems engineer), and went on SS Disability and then Medicare.

My doctor recommended me for LVRS or transplant, so I went to Columbia Presbyterian Hospital for pre-tx testing. This is 3 days of extensive tests to see if you have any health problems, and see if you are healthy enough to survive the surgery, and also to see if you actually need the surgery. They told me my lungs were too far gone for LVRS, and they discovered a major artery was 80% blocked, so I had a stent placed, and went on a year of blood thinners. I also had many of the standard COPD associated diseases: osteoporosis, reflux, high blood pressure, enlarged right side of the heart, arthritis, etc.

Some of this is from the many years of COPD, and some is from the many years of COPD medicine (Prednisone, Albuterol, etc.) I was diagnosed as having "end-stage COPD." I recommend the pre-tx testing to anyone with advanced COPD, whether or not you are interested in transplantation. I never would have known about the blocked artery if I hadn't gone through it.

During the year while I was on blood thinners, and ineligible for transplant, the transplant center put me on the "inactive" transplant list. During this time I was able to spend a year plus in 2-hour education sessions on everything you wanted to know (but were afraid to ask) about respiratory diseases and transplants.

Some examples of the topics included: nutrition, transplant meds, and immunosuppressants, exercise, psychology, finances, Medicare, rejection (acute and chronic), bronchoscopies, external oxygen, survival rates, testing, research, Q&A's, etc., etc., etc.) The education is a requirement to be accepted for transplant. In my center, you are required to attend 10 sessions/year.

I also attended many external seminars, such as World COPD Day all-day seminars and Medicare, Medigap, MAP's, etc.

While you are on the inactive list, you are also tested regularly, to see how close you are to being moved to the "active" list. Once on the "active" list, you can be called at any time they find lungs for you. You can refuse the transplant at any time, even when they call you and tell you they have lungs for you.

Of course, if you refuse, they may not be able to find lungs for you at a later time. All of this time and education can help to let you know if you indeed are   ready (mentally and physically) to have a transplant.

In my tx center, they like to say that they will not put you on the active list unless you are not likely to survive for more than a couple of years without a transplant. Of course, you also have to be healthy enough to survive the surgery. The main criteria are that your survival rate will be better with the surgery than without.

To anyone who might be interested in receiving a transplant, I would like to add that keeping in the best shape that you can, through home exercise or attending pulmonary rehab or PT, is just as important as it is for a COPD patient.

The healthier you are going into surgery, the faster your recovery and the healthier you will be after the surgery.

As for my transplant, once on the active list, I had 3 "dry runs." A dry run is when you get called in (normally in the dead of night, since the hospital that has the donor, normally waits until the end of the day before they call your tx center to come over), and when they check out the lungs, they turn out to be not suitable. This can happen often. Your transplant team cannot know if the donor's lungs are okay until they actually examine the donor and the donor's records.

When I received my first call, I actually was not totally ready to have a transplant. On that day, I felt relatively healthy, and when they told me that the donor's lungs were not suitable, I was happy to go home.

My transplant team actually knew better, however, and knew that I needed the transplant. By the time I got the call, and the donor's lungs were fine, I was totally ready for the tx, and knew I needed it badly. By the way, at the time, I was 58 years old. The surgeon that removed my lungs told me that they were like rocks. I actually did not wait long to be called once I hit the active list. This is because I am relatively tall (6'2"), and most people waiting for lungs are much shorter. (They can't put lungs from a donor over 6' tall into a patient 5'2", or vice versa.)

I definitely know that transplants are not for everyone,

and you are trading one disease for possibly many others due to side effects of all the medications. Kidney disease, diabetes, cancers, etc. are common side effects that many transplant recipients come down with many years after their transplant (not to mention rejection). I can only tell you that right after the tx, I no longer had COPD, I stopped all the COPD medications, inhalers, etc., did away with my wheelchair and oxygen, and am feeling great. I have had a couple of episodes of acute rejection, which is minor and is fixed with a massive dose of prednisone for 3 days, and have had a few other minor problems that only required switching meds until we found the ones that worked for me.

All along, I have not had any breathing problems. As most of you know, there is nothing like not being able to breathe. I consider that the worst!

One thing I DID get from the occasional COPD exacerbations and trips to the local hospital was the ability to cope with the idea of dying. For me, when I could not catch a breath, it prepared me for death. Sorry if that sounds morbid, but it was actually good for me mentally.

Anyway, I'm feeling great and loving life as never before. I have dozens of new friends who have received transplants, and we have regular picnics and parties, and also meet and have lunch when we see each other at the clinic. As a matter of fact, at our holiday party this December, we had a transplant recipient who received a double lung tx in 2002, and just a month before I gave birth to a beautiful new baby boy. What a miracle! Without her tx, she probably would not have even been with us at all, and now she's a new mother. Pretty cool!

And another:

I was perfectly healthy until last August when I had a cold. By Labor Day I was wheezing and on steroids and inhalers for presumed adult-onset asthma. My breathing was getting worse, and evidently, my lungs sounded awful, with little air passing. A CT scan indicated possible emphysema, but I was never a smoker, so this seemed unlikely.

A second opinion at the lung center and it was confirmed that this was neither asthma or emphysema. An open lung biopsy in January confirmed their suspicions; I had Bronchioles Obliterans. I was told the only treatment was a lung transplant. I thought I had a lot of time to get "bad enough" to need a transplant, but I was wrong!

By March I was on 4L oxygen and had to stop working in April. I had the transplant evaluation in early April, was listed in late April. On Friday, May 13th I received a call from UPenn that they had lungs for me. Surgery occurred on Saturday when I received a bilateral lung transplant.

Post-op recovery went very well. I was in the ICU for less than 24 hours and was discharged 9 days later. I probably would have gone home even earlier, but I am now diabetic, and the pulmonary team did not want me to go home on a Friday, so I stayed til Monday and had more education about meds and diabetes. Outpatient rehab started the first-day post op and continued for 3 days/week for 6 weeks.

Since then I have done generally well. I had a problem with severe nausea and vomiting and was re-admitted once for dehydration. Have had some intermittent nausea and vomiting since then, and that seems to be resolved now. I also had a severe drop in my WBC, but after stopping Imuran and 2 doses of Neupogen, my counts have come up, and I am feeling much less fatigued. I am back at work full time (since Jan 2nd), and am finding this to be hard. My brain feels fuzzy at times, which my docs have said may be med related, surgery related, and/or just a normal adjustment to returning to a complex job after being out for almost 10 months.

I am eternally grateful to my donor and his/her family. Their generosity saved my life. I will always be grateful for the wonderful health care team at UPenn. They saved my life, and have supported me along my recovery with care and support. And my family and friends have been amazing!

While all is going rather well, I am struggling with ongoing fatigue. The docs think this may be related to my being over-immunosuppressed, which hopefully is in resolving. Bloods will be checked again in another 2 weeks, and I keep my fingers crossed. Another complication is diabetes. My sugars are well-controlled, but between the diabetes and Prednisone, my weight keeps increasing, which may also be contributing to my fatigue. All of this makes it really difficult to keep up with my exercise routine. I keep pushing out of respect to my donor and myself.

Here is one waiting for the transplant:

My name is Karen R. before February I was a reasonably healthy, stay at home mom of a 2-year-old. In mid-February, I started coughing and becoming short of breath. I immediately went to the doctor and was told I had pneumonia. I was given antibiotics and steroids. I continued to worsen. I was then told I had bronchitis and given more antibiotics and steroids. This went on until I coughed so hard I cracked two ribs and was in unbearable pain.

My next trip was to a Pulmonologist. He took all kinds of X-rays and CAT scans and told me that my sinuses were blocked causing the constant infection. I was put on long-term antibiotics and told I would be better in 6 weeks. By now it is April, and I had been coughing since February. I didn't get any better in the next 6 weeks, so I was hospitalized for testing. A week later — the Friday before Memorial Day weekend — I was diagnosed with BOOP (Bronchiolitis Obliterans Organizing Pneumonia). I was told that with high doses of steroids this would resolve in 6 months to a year.

After 6 months, I was still not getting any better. In fact, my lung function had declined slightly. I was then sent to the Mayo Clinic in for a second opinion. At Mayo, I was told that I had Constrictive Bronchiolitis Obliterans and not BOOP. I was also told that there was very little that could be done to help me. There was no medication that would open up the badly scarred small airways. My only hope was a transplant.

My husband and I were in shock. We had gone to the Mayo Clinic for hope, not devastation. I was not yet 40 years old and in need of an organ transplant. We decided not to believe them and came home determined to find another solution. In January I started seeing an alternative medicine doctor that thought he could help me. After months of treatments, my lung function was still declining, and I was failing physically and emotionally. I finally gave up and made an appointment to see my Pulmonologist to talk to him about transplant. He was very supportive of our decision and made the referral for us at the Cleveland Clinic.

Currently, I am listed for a double lung transplant at the Cleveland Clinic. I have been on the list for over 15 months. I have had one dry run. I am eagerly awaiting the call that will be my gift of life.

The transplant was something that I never thought I would ever have to face in my life, but with the help of my Transplant buddies and my incredible family, I am certain that I have made the right decision. I look forward to that day that I can take a full breath again and dream of the day that I will dance with my son. God Bless!

One more:

My name is Meghann M. I'm 28 years old.

I was a completely normal and healthy kid until I was 12 years old. In February of 1993, I became ill with the Flu. I had all the symptoms and felt crappy. My mom called our family doctor, but his office was full. So, he asked her what my symptoms were over the phone. He said that it sounded like the flu and to just keep treating me with the over the counter medicines. The next day I woke up feeling a lot better and my temperature was gone. I wanted to go to school, but my Mom made me stay home and rest instead. By that evening my temperature was back up to over 101. Plus, I was having trouble breathing. I remember feeling horrible, and I asked her to take me to the ER.

Once at the ER, I was diagnosed with pneumonia in both of my lungs. They put me in the hospital to give me oxygen over night and medicine. During the night, I got worse, and by the next morning, I was in respiratory failure. Our town is small, and they don't even have a pulmonologist on staff. So, they sent me, by ambulance, to the nearest big hospital, which was about 20 minutes away.

Once at the new hospital, I was put on a respirator. The doctors said that I had somehow developed a staph infection on top of the pneumonia and that it was killing all my white blood cells. Therefore, my body was having trouble fighting the infection off. They told my mother that they would do everything they could to save me, but that they couldn't guarantee that I would survive through the night. The staph germ was moving so fast, they didn't know if they would be able to kill it. I had tubes everywhere. Chest tubes, I.V.'s, you name it, I had it.

I was on the respirator for 3 weeks in Pediatric ICU. After they removed me from ICU, I was on the floor for a week, and then they released me from the hospital. Upon my release, the doctors told me that I would have SOME scarring in my lungs from the staph pneumonia, but that it wouldn't be too bad. They said that by the same time next year, I should be recovered enough to do all the things that I had done before I got sick. (i.e. cheerleading, swim team, etc.) And that my life would go back to normal. They sent me home on 1 liter of oxygen with instructions to slowly wean myself off of it.

Trusting that they knew what they were doing, I was slowly weaning my oxygen down. I went for hours during the day without it. But all I could do without it on was just sit still. In addition to that, I was still losing weight even though I was eating like a pig. I had lost down to 85 lbs from 110 lbs, while in the hospital. But, after I got home, I continued to lose weight and got down to as low as 74 pounds. I was a stick. I had no energy. I was pale and looked like a ghost. Concerned, my mother talked to the doctors, and they said that my weight loss was probably because I was depressed and that wasn't eating enough. So, they sent me to a psychiatrist. I was so weak that I couldn't even walk into his office. My step dad had to carry me. The shrink didn't help. All he told me was to treat my food like it was medicine. Yeah, right.

Finally, the pulmonologists at the hospital referred me to Chapel Hill (UNC Hospitals) to visit specialists about my "eating disorder." I went down there that summer in June or July. While I was there, they did a chest x-ray. The doctors were shocked by what they saw. They said my lungs looked like swiss cheese from all the damage to them. Then one day, the transplant surgeon came into my room and looked me in the eye and told me, "With lungs like yours, you won't live longer than 2 years without a transplant." I was horrified. The doctors at Chapel Hill told me that the reason why I kept losing so much weight was not that I wasn't eating enough. It was because my lungs were so damaged that I was using up all my calories just trying to breathe! I was actually doing my body more damage by going without the oxygen. My family and I were in shock. They put me on continuous oxygen at 2 liters at rest and 4 liters with activity. They started the evaluation process, and I was listed that summer.

I waited for over 3 and half years and went through 1 "no-go" (or "dry-run" as some of you call them) while waiting. I have a rare blood type (B +). During this time I went to physical therapy/pulmonary rehab 3 or 4 days a week. I had my teacher bring my work from school to my house. During those 3 and 1/2 years, my lung capacity actually got a little better due to the pulmonary rehab. By the time I was 16, I was able to go out and get around and hang out with my friends. I still had to use my oxygen 24 hours a day, but by that time I was used to it. I decided I wanted to go back to school for as many classes as I could handle. But, I also knew that if I got called for a transplant, I would have to relocate down to Chapel Hill for 3 or 4 months after transplant to do rehab. And that would cause me to miss class, and I wouldn't graduate on time. So, we discussed this with the transplant team, and they told me that I was healthy enough that I could go "inactive" on the list until after I graduated. It was very important to me to go back to school and be with my friends and just try to be as normal a teenager as I could. So, that is what I did.

After HS, I decided that I wanted to go to college. After

meeting with the transplant team again, they actually told me that I was TOO healthy for a transplant right then. And, that I could stay inactive on the list until my lungs got worse or that I was getting closer to needing one. So, I went to college and graduated in Dec. of 2003. I've remained "inactive" on the list for the past 12 years.

But, recently I've been having problems with my CO_2 level staying high, especially at night when I sleep. My pulmonologist recently told me that she felt like I was getting close to having to be reactivated on the list. Before I knew it, I was being scheduled for a re-evaluation; since it had been 15 years since I had my first one. I'm pretty convinced that when the evaluation is over, they are going to reactivate me on the list.

As you read, people are in different stages of the need for a transplant, or they have had it. Some do not live as long as Cody or have a different set of complications. See this story below.

I was diagnosed with Cystic Fibrosis when I was four years old. I lived a very normal childhood despite having to take enzymes with every meal and have chest pt from my mom or dad to help loosen any secretions in my lungs. I started using a nebulizer once a day at the age of 16.

I was first hospitalized at the age of 23 while attending nursing school. I was married a year later and had a daughter Casey at the age of 25. I worked in the nursing field for three years before being diagnosed with a mycobacterium in my lungs. Some of the medications I took for the Mycobacterium gave me toxic hepatitis. It resolved after a couple of weeks, but my weight dropped to 87 lbs. during that time. I received a port soon after diagnosis because I had to receive long-term IV antibiotics.

Over the next year, my lung function fell pretty rapidly, even though I was being treated for the mycobacterium. My doctor then recommended that I start thinking about a lung transplant. My lung function was about 25% when I first started the evaluation for transplant. I was put on oxygen 24/7 at that time.

I was first referred to Barnes-Jewish Hospital in St. Louis but was told there was a 2-year wait for new lungs. Since my doctor didn't think I could wait that long, he then referred me to University Medical Center. After doing some blood work, they found out that I had a large number of antibodies in my blood that made me incompatible with 96% of the population. This meant that it would be very hard to find a cadaver match for me and that I should consider a living-related lobar transplant. In other words, they would start testing family and friends who would be willing to give up a lobe of one of their lungs. They immediately found a match with my Mom's brother. All we had to do was find one more match, and I could receive a transplant. About 40 family members and friends were tested.

While all of these people were being tested, I was going through treatment to try and lower the antibody level in my blood. The lower it went, the better chance I had of finding a donor in time. I had to have Plasmapheresis treatments three times a week at Duke. This treatment is where they remove your blood and separate the plasma from the whole blood to try and remove the circulating antibodies in the plasma. Each treatment lasted about two hours. I then had to get a gamma-globulin infusion which lasted another two hours. The treatment lowered the antibody level some, but not like my physician had hoped. At the same time, I had to have a feeding tube placed through my abdominal wall into my stomach, because I couldn't keep my weight up. The nutritional shakes that I would put through the tube contained so much sugar and carbohydrates that I had to start taking insulin shots. I had to have sinus surgery the same month to try and decrease infection in my sinuses. Because of chronic anemia, I had to have several blood transfusions over the following months.

By September, only one suitable donor had been found,

and my pulmonologist, Dr. P, knew that we needed to find a second donor quickly. My hospitalizations were so frequent at that time that we wondered if we shouldn't just move to the hospital area until transplant. Since we were running out of time, the transplant team decided that my mom should be tested. She wasn't tested before now because she is 3" shorter than I am (donors are supposed to be the same height or taller). She was a match. After going through all of the testings that donors have to go through, they determined that her lungs were actually large for her size. This was a blessing because it meant that her lobe would be of adequate size.

The transplant was scheduled for Oct. 26, 2001. Unfortunately, it had to be canceled because my mom developed a fever the night before surgery. They rescheduled the transplant for Nov. 12, knowing that I didn't have much longer to live.

On Nov. 7, I started running a fever of 103 and was admitted to the hospital. They ran some tests and took some blood cultures to figure out the source of the fever. That night, my blood pressure fell, my pulse rate increased, I had blurred vision, and I became very short of breath. The physician on call had them prepare a room for me in the ICU. By morning, I started feeling better, and by the next afternoon, I was up doing two laps around the hallway. The physician who had been there the night before couldn't believe it. He said he was expecting to find me in ICU hooked up to a ventilator.

The night before the transplant, the blood cultures came back and showed that I had a systemic yeast in my blood. This was so serious that they considered rescheduling the transplant again. Because they knew that I probably wouldn't make it if it was rescheduled, they agreed that the transplant would take place on schedule, and they immediately started me on medication for the infection. At about 6 am, I started getting prepped for surgery, as did my mom and uncle. I had such a peace about me at that time. I remember a little about the OR, but they quickly sedated me. The surgery took about 7 1/2 hours and was performed by Dr. D. My mom and uncle's surgeries took about two hours.

During surgery, the surgeons removed both of my diseased lungs and replaced them with my Mom's left lower lobe and my uncle's right lower lobe. They had to turn the lobes sideways in my chest cavity so that they would fit properly. I now had two beautiful pink lobes that were oxygenating my blood perfectly. The surgeons were very pleased with the surgery and informed my friends and family that everything went well with my surgery and with my mom and uncle's surgeries.

After the transplant, my kidney function declined pretty

rapidly. I gained about 30 lbs of fluid within a week after the transplant. I had to be hospitalized several times within the next several months. I had to have another surgery in December of that year called a Nissen Fundoplication. Since I had reflux, they wanted to stop that with surgery to help prevent rejection of my new lungs. When I wasn't being hospitalized, I was going through rehab to strengthen my new lungs and help recover faster. I was able to leave the hospital and return home 3 months after transplant. What a great day that was. My kidney function was close to normal again, and I was feeling great.

A lot has happened since February 2002. First of all, my lung capacity exceeded what they thought it would, so that has been great. I have also been able to keep my weight up for the most part. I have had many hospitalizations for my chronic sinus infections and had my third sinus surgery. I have also been hospitalized for my diabetes. They found a mycobacterium in my lungs 3 months post-transplant, but that seems to have disappeared with medication. I continue to be deaf in my left ear and partially deaf in my right due to all of the IV antibiotics I was on pre-transplant. They thought that after I went off of the IV meds, some of my hearing would return, but unfortunately, it hasn't. Because of the prednisone that I have been taking since transplant, I have severe osteoporosis in my lumbar spine. I have had 2 more blood clots which have resolved, and I am currently dealing with some chronic rejection that is being treated with an increase in anti-rejection meds. My kidneys aren't doing so well (the meds, high b.p. and the diabetes has taken a toll on them). I am currently being evaluated for a kidney transplant. *Due to all her complications, she passed.*

+++

I could go on forever telling stories of success and failures. However, while I was in the hospital waiting on Cody, many patients received Kidneys, Liver and other types of transplants. Colorado University works on the wounded vets that have returned from many of the war-torn countries. I saw them replace their hands, legs and even a portion of a face. Many of them burn victims. I would go home crying, seeing these young people so severely injured. We are so blessed with our medical knowledge and how it has affected so many lives in so many positive ways.

+++

Everyone who has had a transplant of some kind reacts differently, some have a single transplant, some receive a heart. Some that I have talked to were out of the hospital in a week, we were not that lucky. I have not found anyone that went through what Cody did, so we were blessed he survived.

NOTE: Additional Information

University of Colorado Hospital is named among the top 10 academic hospitals in the United States, U.S. News & World Report ranks the University of Colorado Hospital as the best in the state.

University HealthSystem Consortium's full list of 2015 winners:

NYU Langone Medical Center

Rush University Medical Center

Mayo Clinic Hospital – Rochester

Emory University Hospital

Froedtert & the Medical College of Wisconsin Hospital

University of Colorado Hospital (UCHealth)

University of Utah Health Care

Houston Methodist Hospital

The Ohio State University-Wexner Medical Center

Memorial Hermann-Texas Medical Center

Beaumont Hospital – Royal Oak

Tufts Medical Center

The University of Kansas Hospital Authority

Some of the Sources for the story:

1. American College of Chest Physicians. A Guide to Lung Transplantation. Available from: http://www.chestnet.org/education/patient/guides/transplantation/index.php.

2. United Network for Organ Sharing. Organ Procurement and Transplantation Network. Available from: http://www.unos.org/data/default.asp?displayType=us Datahttp://www.unos.org/data/default.asp?displayType =usData.

3. American College of Chest Physicians. A Guide to Lung Transplantation. Available from: http://www.chestnet.org/education/patient/guides/tran splantation/index.php.

4. American Thoracic Society. International Guidelines for the Selection of Lung Transplant Candidate. American Journal of Respiratory and Critical Care Medicine 1998. Vol. 158: 335-339.

5. Scientific Registry of Transplant Recipients. Fast Facts About Transplants for 2003. Available from: http://www.ustransplant.org/scr_0704/facts.phphttp:// www.ustransplant.org/scr_0704/facts.php.

6. Scientific Registry of Transplant Recipients. Transplant Primer: Section 5 Lung Transplant 2004. Available from: http://www.ustransplant.org/lung_primer.phphttp://ww w.ustransplant.org/lung_primer.php.

7. American College of Chest Physicians. A Guide to Lung Transplantation. Available from: http://www.chestnet.org/education/patient/guides/tran

splantation/index.php.

8. United Network for Organ Sharing. Organ Procurement and Transplantation Network. Available from: http://www.unos.org/data/default.asp?displayType=us Datahttp://www.unos.org/data/default.asp?displayType =usData.

9. Scientific Registry of Transplant Recipients. Transplant Primer: Section 5 Lung Transplant 2004. Available from: http://www.ustransplant.org/lung_primer.php.

Medline Plus. Lung Transplant. Available from:

10. http://www.nlm.nih.gov/medlineplus/ency/article/0030 10.htmhttp://www.nlm.nih.gov/medlineplus/ency/articl e/003010.htm.

11. United Network for Organ Sharing. Organ Procurement and Transplantation Network. Available from: http://www.unos.org/data/default.asp?displayType=us Data.

View projects funded by the American Lung Association for 2004-2005

Medications for Lung Transplant Patients:

After a lung transplant, patients are generally given drugs that will suppress the body's natural immune system. This is to prevent the body from rejecting the new lungs. A strict medication regimen needs to be followed after lung transplantation to ensure the survival of the transplanted lungs and the health of the patient.

Types of Medications:

Immunosuppressant Drugs - these drugs suppress the immune system. They need to be administered to prevent organ rejections.

Anti-infective Drugs - these drugs need to be administered to prevent infection caused by a lowered immune system.

Anti-hypertensive Drugs - these drugs may need to be taken because hypertension may be a side effect of immunosuppressive treatment.

Supplements - these may be recommended by your transplant physician.

Some Do's and Don'ts of Medication

DO:

Learn all the names of your medicines

Take all the medication as ordered

Keep your medications in a dry place, away from heat or direct sunlight

Report any side effects to the transplant coordinator or your transplant physician

If you are uncertain about a medication or dosage, call the transplant coordinator

DON'T:

Do not double the next dose if you miss a dose. Take the next dose as ordered.

Do not take any medications not prescribed by your transplant physician. This includes over the counter drugs.

Always check with your transplant coordinator or physician to see if the medications are permissible.

Immunosuppressant Drugs:

Cyclosporine - Cyclosporine is taken to prevent rejection of the lungs and has greatly increased the survival of all transplant patients. It is best not to miss a dose of this medication. Do not stop taking cyclosporine for any reason without the approval of your transplant physician. Some side effects may include headaches and tremors. Cyclosporine may also cause increase hair growth.

Tacrolimus - Tacrolimus is an alternative drug that may be used to prevent rejection. As with Cyclosporine, you should do your best to not miss a dosage. The side effects are else headaches and tremors. Tacrolimus can also cause high potassium levels.

Azathioprine - It is used in conjunction with your other anti-rejection medications. Azathioprine has relatively few side effects. In rare cases, it may cause liver and pancreas abnormalities.

Mycophenolic Acid - Mycophenolic acid may be used instead of azathioprine in conjunction with other drugs.

Prednisone - Prednisone is a steroid similar to what the adrenal gland normally produces. Prednisone should not be skipped. Prednisone, an appetite stimulant, can lead to overeating and cause cosmetic changes. The most serious of these is weight gain occurring mostly in the trunk. The face may become rounded (moon face) and a fat pad may develop between the shoulder blades. You may develop acne on the face or back; treat with over-the-counter acne medications. Your skin may become oily and hair growth more prominent. Women who are concerned about this may use over the counter bleaching agents. Over time your skin may become thin and bruise easily.

Prednisone causes salt and water retention which may result in swollen ankles and increased blood pressure. You may notice a weakness in your leg muscles. It is important to maintain good muscle tone by exercising daily.

Symptoms will decrease as the drug's dose is decreased over time. Over time prednisone frequently causes bone thinning and your bones may become more brittle. You may be advised to take medications to prevent osteoporosis. Some patients taking prednisone for a prolonged period of time develop cataracts; schedule periodic eye exams. Prednisone may aggravate pre-existing diabetes or unmask latent diabetes.

Sirolimus - Sirolimus is an immunosuppressive agent, although its use is much less than the others listed above.

Anti-infective Drugs

Co-Trimoxazole - This is a combination drug that prevents infections involving the lung and urinary tract. Tell your physician if you are allergic to sulfa drugs because other drugs can be used.

Valcyte - Valcyte is an antiviral medication given to prevent cytomegalovirus (CMV). Your complete blood count and kidney function tests will be closely monitored while you are on this medication. The most frequent side effect of the drug being lowering of white blood count and platelet count.

Ganciclovir - Ganciclovir is an antiviral medication given to prevent and treat cytomegalovirus (CMV). It is administered the first three months intravenously to lung transplants. An oral formulation may be given after the IV course.

Acyclovir - Acyclovir is used to prevent and treat herpes infections. It is used to treat skin, lip, and genital herpes infections as well as shingles.

Itraconazole - Itraconazole is prescribed for the prevention and treatment of certain fungal infections.

Voriconazole - Voriconazole is used like itraconazole to prevent and treat certain fungal infections.

Nystatin - Nystatin is used to prevent and treat yeast and fungal infections involving the mouth, throat, and esophagus and to treat skin, nail, and vaginal fungal infections. Take the ordered dose and swish it inside the mouth for several minutes before swallowing.

Clotrimazole - Clotrimazole is prescribed for candida infections of the mouth (thrush). Either nystatin or clotrimazole usually is prescribed for approximately one month after transplant. It also will be used if the patient develops thrush at some later date.

Anti-hypertensive Drugs

There is a large range of drugs here. It may be more useful to look at this as a concept rather than a list of medications.

Beta and Alpha Blockers - Beta blockers and alpha blockers (clonidine) are additional classes which are typically used in transplant patients as well.

Calcium Channel Blockers - Some of the calcium channel blockers interact with cyclosporine. Therefore, it is important that only your transplant physician change the dose of these medicines.

Diuretics - Diuretics must be used only under supervision. Diuretics are prescribed to help reduce fluid buildup. They cause the kidneys to eliminate excess water and salt from the body into the urine and are used to treat swelling water retention as well as high blood pressure.

Supplements

Calcium - Calcium may be taken by transplant patients because some transplant medications such as prednisone, cyclosporine, and diuretics lead to calcium loss and cause osteoporosis and bone loss.

Magnesium - A magnesium supplement may be ordered due to therapy depleting it. A low magnesium level can cause irritability, muscle weakness, cramps, tingling and irregular heartbeats. Take it with meals; taken on an empty stomach magnesium may cause diarrhea.

+++

These statistics are based on data from 2008. The source data made no distinction between living and deceased donor organs, nor was any distinction made between lobar, single, and double lung transplants.

	1 year survival	5 year survival	10 year survival
Lung transplant	83.6%	53.4%	28.4%
Heart-lung transplant	73.8%	46.5%	28.3%

Transplanted lungs typically last three to five years before showing signs of failure.

Because of all the medication, Kidney disease can occur, here is some information on that possibility. Thank goodness Cody does not have that yet.

"The advent of cyclosporine revolutionized solid organ transplantation and made lung transplantation a clinical reality. Cyclosporine and tacrolimus are calcineurin inhibitors, and they inhibit the proliferation of the primary immune cells responsible for rejection after organ transplantation. Prior to the introduction of cyclosporine, high doses of prednisone were necessary to reduce the risk of rejection. In the early 1980s, surgical techniques were refined, and the introduction of cyclosporine allowed the prevention of rejection, making clinical lung transplantation a reality. Tacrolimus was then introduced in the 1990s and has been shown to be modestly superior to cyclosporine in preventing rejection. Unfortunately, however, both drugs have some potentially serious side effects that can be essentially unavoidable. Obviously, as immunosuppressants, they can predispose to opportunistic infections and even increase the risk of cancer since the immune system plays a role in detecting and inhibiting the proliferation of pre-cancers. Furthermore, both cyclosporine and tacrolimus can cause high blood pressure and kidney disease. They constrict the arteries supplying blood to the kidneys and reduce overall blood flow to the kidneys. They can also lead to progressive kidney scarring over time. In the early stages, the kidney injury is completely reversible, but over time, chronic kidney damage becomes irreversible.

Chronic kidney disease is typically asymptomatic until the late stages. The serum creatinine is a rough estimate of kidney function that is somewhat dependent on age, gender, body size, and muscle mass. Before transplantation, the serum creatinine is usually normal reflecting normal kidney function, but it often begins to rise and reach abnormally high levels in the first year after transplantation. This mild degree of abnormal kidney function is not usually associated with any physical signs or symptoms. Indeed, kidney disease progresses silently until advanced stages. Some of the earliest overt physical signs of kidney disease include fluid retention and high blood pressure; the serum creatinine is usually abnormal at this stage. As the kidney disease progresses, fluid retention and high blood pressure become more difficult to control, but other symptoms are usually absent until kidney failure is imminent. Symptoms of kidney failure include nausea, anorexia, fatigue, weight loss, and shortness of breath with activities as the lungs become congested with fluid.

Approximately 25% of patients have an abnormal serum creatinine within one year of lung transplantation. At this stage, most patients have few symptoms related to their kidney disease. However, 1-2% of patients develop kidney failure requiring dialysis within one year; these patients have typically suffered severe kidney injury in the immediate post-operative recovery period after the transplant. Within five years of transplantation, approximately 35% of patients have an abnormal serum creatinine, and 3-4% are on dialysis or have had a kidney transplant. Clearly, kidney failure is a serious problem after lung transplantation, and its complications can seriously jeopardize the outcome.

Unfortunately, there are few interventions to slow the progression of kidney disease since cyclosporine and tacrolimus are the primary causes. The primary approach has been to target lower blood levels of the drugs when a patient develops kidney disease, but this can sometimes be difficult when managing rejection. In some patients who have had little or no rejection, but have developed early kidney disease, substituting sirolimus for cyclosporine or tacrolimus may be a viable option. Sirolimus, by itself, is not nephrotoxic, but when used in combination with cyclosporine or tacrolimus can worsen the kidney disease. So, some patients can be managed with a combination of sirolimus, prednisone, and azathioprine or mycophenolate mofetil. However, sirolimus is not a panacea; it has multiple side effects that often limit its use, including fluid retention, nausea, diarrhea, low white blood cell count, and it can rarely injure the lungs.

In addition, lung function needs to be carefully monitored when a patient is managed with a drug combination that does not include cyclosporine or tacrolimus since some patients have developed late rejection on this combination. Since there is little latitude to adjust the immunosuppressive regimen to mitigate the progression of kidney disease, optimal control of other risk factors such as diabetes and high blood pressure become paramount. In addition, avoiding other medicines that can be toxic to the kidneys, such as non-steroidal anti-inflammatory drugs like ibuprofen, is also very important.

Unfortunately, kidney disease is a common complication after lung transplantation because of the necessary immunosuppressive regimen. Clearly, this has an adverse impact on quality of life and survival after transplantation, but hopefully, the progression of kidney disease can be prevented as new immunosuppressive regimens become available."

+++

Regardless of the outcomes, a transplant of any type gives life to an individual who needs it, whether it is for one year or twenty. They are blessed because of donors and donor families. Thank you as a donor for giving the greatest gift...life.

www.ingramcontent.com/pod-product-compliance
Lightning Source LLC
Chambersburg PA
CBHW062001280526
45787CB00005B/1950